KU-102-098

School Health, Nutrition and Education for All

Levelling the Playing Field

Matthew C. H. Jukes

Lesley J. Drake

Donald A. P. Bundy

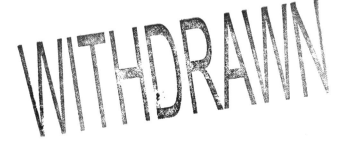

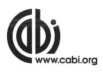

www.cabi.org

LIVERPOOL JMU LIBRARY

3 1111 01449 2233

CABI Publishing is a division of CAB International

CABI Publishing
CAB International
Wallingford
Oxfordshire OX10 8DE
UK
Tel: +44 (0)1491 832111
Fax: +44 (0)1491 833508
E-mail: cabi@cabi.org
Website: www.cabi-publishing.org

CABI Publishing
875 Massachusetts Avenue
7th Floor
Cambridge, MA 02139
USA
Tel: +1 617 395 4056
Fax: +1 617 354 6875
E-mail: cabi-nao@cabi.org

©CAB International 2008. All rights reserved. No part of this publication may be reproduced in any form or by any means, electronically, mechanically, by photocopying, recording or otherwise, without the prior permission of the copyright owners.

A catalogue record for this book is available from the British Library, London, UK.

Library of Congress Cataloging-in-Publication Data

Jukes, Matthew C. H.
 School health, nutrition and education for all : levelling the playing field / Matthew
C.H. Jukes, Lesley J. Drake, Donald A.P. Bundy.
    p. ; cm.
 Includes bibliographical references and index.
 ISBN 978-1-84593-311-1 (alk. paper)
 1.   School children--Health and hygiene--Developing countries. 2. Children Nutrition--
Developing countries. I. Drake, Lesley J. II. Bundy, Donald A. P. III. Title.
 [DNLM: 1. School Health Services--utilization. 2. Child. 3. Developing Countries. 4. Educational
Status. 5. Health Promotion. 6. Nutrition Policy. WA 350 J93s 2007]

 LB3409.D44J85 2007
 371.7'16091724--dc22

                                                                                2007017753

ISBN   978 1 84593 311 1

Printed and bound in the UK from copy supplied by the authors by Biddles Ltd, King's Lynn.

Contents

List of boxes, figures and tables

Boxes

Figures

Tables

List of abbreviations and acronyms

ACT	Artemisinin-based combination therapy
AIDS	Acquired Immune Deficiency Syndrome
ARI	Acute respiratory infection
ARTIs	Acute respiratory tract infections
ARV	Antiretroviral
CBO	Community-Based Organisation
CEE	Central and Eastern Europe
CIS	Commonwealth of Independent States
CRS	Congenital rubella syndrome
DALYs	Disability adjusted life years
DFID	United Kingdom's Department for International Development
DQ	Development quotient
ECD	Early Child Development
EFA	Education for All
FBO	Faith-Based Organisation
FRESH	Focusing Resources on Effective School Health
GER	Gross enrolment ratio
HIV	Human Immunodeficiency Virus
IDA	Iron deficiency anaemia
IDD	Iodine deficiency disorders
IEC	Information education and communication
IMCI	Integrated Management of Childhood Illness
INGO	International Non-Governmental Organisation
IPT	Intermittent preventive treatment
IQ	Intelligence quotient
LBW	Low birth weight
LRTIs	Lower respiratory tract infections
MDGs	Millennium Development Goals
MoH	Ministry of Health
MTCT	Mother-to-child transmission
NGO	Non-Governmental Organisation

OECD	Organisation for Economic Co-operation and Development
OME	Otitis media with effusion
OR	Odds ratio
PCD	Partnership for Child Development
PPC	Partners for Parasite Control
PROGRESA	Programa de Educación, Salud y Alimentación (Mexico)
PTA	Parent Teacher Association
SD	Standard deviation
SEECALINE II	Surveillance et Education des Ecoles et des Communautés en matière d'Alimentation et de Nutrition Elargie, Phase II
SGA	Small for gestational age
STIs	Sexually transmitted infections
UN	United Nations
UNAIDS	Joint United Nations Programme on HIV&AIDS
UNESCO	United Nations Educational Scientific and Cultural Organisation
UNICEF	United Nations Children's Fund
UTIs	Urinary tract infections
WFP	World Food Programme
WHA	World Health Assembly of WHO
WHO	World Health Organisation

Acknowledgements

This book has benefited from discussions with several colleagues during the writing of a previous chapter on "School-Based Health and Nutrition Programs" in the book *Disease Control Priorities in Developing Countries*[1]. We would like to thank Kathleen Beegle, Sheldon Shaeffer, Amaya Gillespie, Seung-hee Frances Lee, Anna-Maria Hoffman, Jack Jones, Arlene Mitchell, Delia Barcelona, Balla Camara, Chuck Golmar, Lorenzo Savioli, Malick Sembene, Tsutomu Takeuchi and Cream Wright for their valuable contributions in this regard.

We are very grateful to Criana Connal for comments on drafts of the book and to Dick Murnane for cleaning up our imprecise use of terminology from the field of Economics.

We would like to thank Anastasia Said for tireless editing work and to thank both Richard Suswillo at the Partnership for Child Development (PCD) and Sarah Hulbert at CAB International for smoothing the process of manuscript completion.

---

[1] Jamison, D.T., J.G. Breman, A.R. Measham, G. Alleyne, M. Claeson, D.B. Evans, P. Jha, A. Mills, P. Musgrove, *Disease control priorities in developing countries*. Second Edition. 2006, New York: Oxford University Press.

About the authors

Matthew Jukes is Assistant Professor of Education at the Harvard Graduate School of Education. He was trained in developmental psychology at the University of Oxford and has since conducted research on education and child development throughout Africa and South Asia. He was previously based at the Partnership for Child Development, Imperial College, London; the Institute of Education in London; and at Yale University.

Lesley Drake has a PhD in parasitology and is the Director of the Partnership for Child Development (PCD), based at the Department of Infectious Disease Epidemiology, Imperial College School of Medicine, London. Created in 1992, PCD is an organisation that works with civil society and international aid agencies to turn the findings of evidence-based research into national, large-scale school health and nutrition programmes. Her main focus is to coordinate teams providing technical support to governments of low income countries in the design, implementation and evaluation of school health, nutrition and HIV&AIDS programmes. See http://www.schoolsandhealth.org/.

Donald Bundy is the Lead Specialist on school health, nutrition and HIV&AIDS at the World Bank and currently provides technical and operational support to school health, nutrition and HIV&AIDS programmes globally. Previously a Professor of Epidemiology at the University of Oxford and the Director of PCD, he has contributed to many of the studies quoted in this book. He is the author of *Education and HIV/AIDS: A Window of Hope* and more than 300 other school health and nutrition related publications. He was a co-founder of the partnership on Focusing Resources on Effective School Health (FRESH).

About the book

"A major step forward in building the argument for school health and nutrition and Education for All."

Francisco Espejo,
Chief School Feeding Service,
World Food Programme

"Persuasively argues that moderate investment in school health and nutrition programmes now will reap great dividends for hundreds of millions of children, for their education and for their future after school."

David Bloom,
Clarence James Gamble Professor of Economics and Demography,
Harvard School of Public Health

Chapter 1

The compelling case for school health and nutrition

Challenges in achieving Education for All

Providing education to children is not a simple task. For children to benefit from a full course of primary education, many things need to be in place: a school that provides the essential materials required for learning and a motivated and well trained teacher guided by strong school leadership. Children need to learn free from competing distractions in the home. Families need to find other ways and means to carry out responsibilities traditionally falling to children and they need to provide money for uniforms, school equipment and in some cases school fees too. Children need to be supported by caregivers who understand the process of education and encourage children in their efforts. Girls in particular need to be given every opportunity to do well and the support to take these opportunities. Children themselves need to be motivated to succeed; they need to see the rewards for their efforts in the availability of secondary school places and in jobs and livelihoods that reward the investment in their education. All these things need to be in place for children to develop essential skills from a full course of primary education, and not just for 1 day or 2 days or a week, but for every day of every school term for 6, 7 or 8 years. Considering the complexity and scale of the task involved, it is perhaps not surprising that global and national efforts, supported by years of development assistance have yet to fulfil the promise of Education for All (EFA).

Education for All is a global movement committed to achieving six goals agreed in the 2000 Dakar Framework for Action. This book looks at how improving children's health and nutrition is essential for reaching these goals. In particular it is concerned with the ultimate goals of promoting access and

©CAB International 2008. *School Health, Nutrition and Education for All:* 1
Levelling the Playing Field (M.C.H. Jukes *et al.*)

**Box 1.1. The Dakar Education for All Goals and
the UN Millennium Development Goals**

The Dakar Education for All Goals

The goals establish a framework for action that is designed to enable all individuals to realise their right to learn and to fulfil their responsibility to contribute to the development of their society.

(i) Expanding and improving comprehensive early childhood care and education, especially for the most vulnerable and disadvantaged children;

(ii) ensuring that by 2015 all children, particularly girls, children in difficult circumstances and those belonging to ethnic minorities, have access to and complete free and compulsory primary education of good quality;

(iii) ensuring that the learning needs of all young people and adults are met through equitable access to appropriate learning and life skills programmes;

(iv) achieving a 50 per cent improvement in levels of adult literacy by 2015, especially for women, and equitable access to basic and continuing education for all adults;

(v) eliminating gender disparities in primary and secondary education by 2005, and achieving gender equality in education by 2015, with a focus on ensuring girls' full and equal access to and achievement in basic education of good quality;

(vi) improving all aspects of the quality of education and ensuring excellence of all so that recognised and measurable learning outcomes are achieved by all, especially in literacy, numeracy and essential life skills.

The UN Millennium Development Goals

Of the eight Millennium Development Goals approved by world leaders at the United Nations Millennium Summit in 2000, Goals 2 and 3 focus on education explicitly while education is an essential part of achieving Goal 1.

Goal 1: Eradicate extreme poverty and hunger
- Reduce by half the proportion of people living on less than a dollar a day
- Reduce by half the proportion of people who suffer from hunger

Goal 2: Achieve universal primary education
- Ensure that all boys and girls complete a full course of primary education

Goal 3: Promote gender equality and empower women
- Eliminate gender disparity in primary and secondary education, preferably by 2005, and at all levels by 2015

Source: UNESCO (2000)[1], United Nations (2001)[2].

achievement in primary schools, and with school health and nutrition programmes that can be delivered through the primary school system. As such we are most concerned with EFA goals 2, 5 and 6, which address issues of access, gender equity and the quality of basic education, and map onto the two education-related Millennium Development Goals (see Box 1.1). So, what progress has been made towards these goals? By 2004, 86 per cent of school-age children were attending primary schools worldwide. In the 5 year period to 2004, enrolments grew by 27 per cent in sub-Saharan Africa and by 19 per cent in South and West Asia. However, many challenges remain. There are still 77 million out of school at the primary level. The proportion of enrolled children who complete primary education is less than two-thirds in most countries in sub-Saharan Africa and little higher in South and West Asia. The target for eliminating gender disparities in education by 2005 has already been missed. Although progress has been made – there are now 94 girls attending school for every 100 boys, compared to a figure of 92, 5 years ago – there is a concern that the countries where gender disparities are greatest are the ones making the slowest progress. In short, access, quality, completion rates and gender equity remain a problem. There are many challenges ahead.

School health and nutrition: a "quick win"

From the perspective of an educator, health initiatives can seem like simple affairs. In contrast with the sustained and complex effort required to teach basic skills to a child, vaccinations, for example, can deliver lifelong protection from disease in a matter of minutes. Health initiatives are, of course, not without their own set of challenges. But the comparison between the long-term benefits of short intensive vaccination campaigns and the persistent daily efforts of teachers and pupils towards educational achievement is one way to understand why the major achievements of development assistance have been in global health. The elimination of smallpox from the world and of poliomyelitis (polio) in the Americas, dramatic reductions in measles infection and the prevention of diarrhoeal diseases are some of the reasons why children are now twice as likely to survive to age 5, than they were 50 years ago. If only the world of education could replicate this success. But education cannot be delivered in a single shot or a course of pills. There is no short-cut to a quality education.

Well, no. But school health and nutrition programmes are a way to apply the simple effectiveness of global health interventions to deliver large gains in education. This book will argue that poor health and nutrition are major barriers to educational access and achievement among poor communities. The vast number of children living with diseases like malaria, worm infections and iron deficiency anaemia and the substantial impact these diseases have on education, draws attention to school health and nutrition as an issue of great importance. The simple and highly cost-effective methods for treating these diseases, through school-based health services, make the issue an urgent education policy priority for all poor countries. School health and nutrition programmes are clearly a "quick win"[3] in the efforts towards Education for All.

Levelling the playing field

A major attraction of school health and nutrition programmes is that they do something that few other education interventions do: they have the greatest benefit for the poorest children. To understand why that is the case, we need to invoke the concepts of Double Jeopardy and Capability Theory.

The Double Jeopardy of disease among the poor

Taking these concepts one at a time, Double Jeopardy was originally applied to at-risk children in the United States[4] but for our purposes refers to the way in which the poorest in society suffer twice at the hands of disease and poor nutrition. The first way in which the poor are in jeopardy is by being more likely to suffer a condition of poor health or poor nutrition. Without exception, the diseases that affect children and their education are most prevalent in poor countries and in the poorest communities within those countries. The most striking statistic is that 99 per cent of child deaths occur in poor countries. This picture of inequality is the same when looking at the diseases of concern in this book – those that rarely kill but do impair the quality of life and of learning for millions of children. This brings us to the second way in which the poor are in jeopardy – conditions of poor health and nutrition have the biggest educational impact on the poor. That is, even when disease reaches rich and poor alike, the poor are most likely to experience disruption to their learning as a result. This differential impact happens because the poor have less capacity to cope with the additional burden of a new disease. Already struggling to pursue their education in the face of poverty, delayed development and poor general health, the marginal impact of a new infection or a nutritional disease can push them over the edge. They don't have the financial, physical or mental resources to cope. Double Jeopardy is the unacceptable state of the world's poor but it is also the hopeful message of school health and nutrition: delivering simple and effective treatment to children in schools brings double benefits to the poor and a big step towards equity in educational outcomes.

School health and nutrition programmes develop capabilities

Another way of understanding how school health and nutrition programmes promote equity is through Capability Theory. In his influential account of this theory, Amartya Sen[5] argues that development should be a process of expanding people's capabilities to pursue a life that they have reason to value. This contrasts with resource-based views of development, which promote expansion of available resources, such as income. One of the arguments for a focus on capabilities rather than resources is based on equity. Individuals differ in their ability to utilise resources. Those who are disadvantaged, for example, through disease or disability, require additional resources to achieve the same ends as others who are not so disadvantaged. Thus, an equal distribution of resources does not guarantee an equality of outcomes. When extra resources are provided, they bring greater benefits to those who are most capable and in this way can serve to exacerbate inequalities. On the other hand, a focus on the development of capabilities leads to improved, and more equally distributed abilities to utilise resources.

This abstract argument takes form in its application to educational interventions. Some efforts to improve education involve providing additional resources. For example, a policy or project may aim to improve the quality of education by distributing textbooks to children. In such circumstances, children differ in their capabilities to benefit from the additional resources. Some children can read better than others; some have existing knowledge that may help them to understand the book's contents; some are healthier and thus better able to concentrate when reading. In this way, the more capable – the richer, smarter, healthier children – benefit the most and inequalities are widened. This theoretical position is borne out by evidence. From textbook provision[6] to teacher incentives[7], educational interventions bring the greatest benefits to the highest achieving children. Wherever differential impacts are documented, inequalities increase.

From this viewpoint, school health and nutrition programmes can be seen as interventions to expand capabilities rather than to increase resources. Improved health improves children's capabilities to benefit from education. Furthermore, the capabilities of the poorest, and usually least capable students, are improved to the greatest extent. This helps to promote equity in the classroom. Note also, that when a more equal distribution of capabilities is achieved, further investments in resources, such as the provision of new textbooks, will benefit children more equally. When the inequality of capabilities is reduced, so too are inequalities in the use of resources. Disadvantaged children are more likely to benefit from new textbooks when they have the capabilities to do so – the ability to concentrate that comes with good health and the necessary reading skills and knowledge. Thus, school health and nutrition programmes have the greatest benefits for the poorest children and also increase the likelihood that further improvements in educational quality will bring benefits to all. Capability Theory helps explain why school health and nutrition is such a powerful tool for levelling the playing field.

Developing the case for school health and nutrition

The arguments above represent the central thesis of this book. Tough challenges remain in the Education for All movement; school health and nutrition programmes offer a "quick win" in attempts to address these challenges because health and nutrition can be improved cost-effectively and because doing so bring large benefits for children's education. School health and nutrition programmes help promote equity because they relieve the poor of the Double Jeopardy of higher prevalence and greater educational impact of disease and because they develop the capabilities to benefit from educational resources. However, there are more elements to the case for school health and nutrition. School health and nutrition programmes owe their effectiveness to the confluence of many aspects of disease and its impact on education (see Box 1.2 for use of the term 'disease' throughout this book). This section sets out these elements of the case for school health and nutrition and outlines how they are developed throughout the book.

Box 1.2. What is a disease?

Disease is defined as:

"an abnormal condition of the body or part of it, arising from any cause"[8].

Thus, disease can have its origins in any cause from genetics to parasitic infections. We use this broad definition of disease in part to cover conditions of ill health due to poor nutrition as well as to infection. The programmes discussed in this book intentionally include the terms 'health' and 'nutrition' in order to associate them with work in two distinct fields: those working in global health and largely focusing on infectious disease, and those working in nutritional sciences. Our broad use of the term 'disease' is designed to include both of these fields.

Moreover, disease is not restricted to conditions associated with poverty. It is increasingly recognised that many developing countries suffer the "double burden of disease"[9]. Such countries are increasingly affected by diseases traditionally associated with affluence, such as obesity, while still struggling to combat the diseases of poverty, such as infectious disease and undernutrition.

Chapter 2 is concerned with challenges to child health and nutrition. We discussed above why the success of global health initiatives, such as immunisation programmes, are difficult to replicate in the field of education. Such global health initiatives provide a motivation for school health and nutrition programmes in another way. The success in reducing child mortality means that many more children are surviving into the school-age years. Now, attention is turning to the quality of the life these children lead and their ability to benefit from education. Many of the diseases these children suffer may affect their learning. If this is the case, it is a concern because **diseases that affect education are highly prevalent.** The numbers are staggering. To take just one example, the number of people with worm infections worldwide runs into the billions. Roughly one-third of all schoolchildren are infected with these worms, one-half stunted in growth due to poor nutrition and a third have iron deficiency anaemia. These diseases rarely kill, but the effect they have on education is replicated on a colossal scale. The cumulative damage is incalculable (although we do make an attempt to calculate it in Chapter 6).

The distribution of these diseases is as big a concern as their prevalence. Efforts to increase access to education often fail at the final hurdle. Reaching the final 10 per cent, the poorest and most vulnerable, presents the biggest challenge. So it is a concern that poor health and nutrition are additional barriers to education for these children because **the poor are more likely to suffer from poor health and nutrition.** This is true for preschool children who account for more than 50 per cent of the global gap in mortality between the poorest and richest quintiles of the world's population and they bear 30 per cent of the total burden of disease in poor countries. It is also true for school-age children. Inequalities persist.

The good news is that something can be done about this situation. There is great potential for interventions to improve the conditions of the poor **because diseases that affect education are preventable and treatable.** In many cases, the treatment of these diseases is simple and effective. Intestinal worms can be removed with a single pill given biannually. Iron deficiency anaemia can be controlled through weekly supplementation with pills containing iron compounds. Much can be done to prevent malaria infection through the use of insecticide treated bednets or intermittent preventive treatment for mothers and infants.

As children grow, the health and nutritional challenges they face change. For infants, diarrhoeal diseases present the largest threat. Throughout early childhood cerebral malaria is most significant. By the time children are in school, worm infections become a major cause of disease. Most of the illness resulting from worm infections is suffered by schoolchildren. Similarly, a large proportion of undernutrition and anaemia is suffered by schoolchildren. In general we find that **schoolchildren bear the greatest burden of some of the most common diseases that affect education.** This means that programmes to reach school-age children can have a large impact on the global prevalence of these diseases and the illness caused by them. This is the final of four main conclusions to be drawn from Chapter 2.

Chapters 3 to 5 assess the impact of health and nutrition on education. This survey of research demonstrates the numerous ways in which education can be affected by health and nutrition. *Chapter 3* looks at access to education, including issues of enrolment, drop-out and absenteeism. There are many ways in which access to education is affected by poor health and nutrition. Some diseases have severe effects on children's development and consequently their chances of enrolment. Polio infection can lead to physical disability and iodine deficiency can lead to severe mental retardation. In both cases, poor countries are less likely to have the facilities to provide education to children with such disabilities. Less severe diseases have effects on school enrolment too. Malaria infection can decrease a girl's likelihood of going to school. Short stature due to poor nutritional status can lead parents to delay children's enrolment. Once children are enrolled in school, illness due to malaria or worm infections, for example, can cause children to miss school.

Chapter 4 looks at the long-term effects of early childhood illness on educational achievement. There are many ways in which these long-term effects can occur. For example, poorly nourished young children are less sociable, more apathetic and generally less likely to interact with their environment. Responding to their apathy, mothers are less likely to interact with poorly nourished children. This lack of stimulation from the environment can affect children's mental development. In addition, malaria, iron deficiency and undernutrition have direct effects on the brain. Suffering from these diseases in early childhood has a long-term impact on cognitive development into adolescence.

Chapter 5 considers the evidence that children's learning suffers from poor health and nutrition while they are at school. Cognitive abilities in this age group are poorer among children who miss breakfast and who have malaria, worm infections, or iron deficiency. Treating children for these diseases can improve their potential to learn, but there is a need for quality education to help children exploit this potential.

Several conclusions can be drawn from the review of evidence in Chapters 3 to 5. One conclusion is that **disease affects education throughout childhood.** Education can be affected by disease prenatally, in infancy, in early childhood or in the school-age years. Interventions are required at all stages of this process. A life cycle approach to disease control is required through programmes of maternal child health, the Integrated Management of Childhood Illness (IMCI), Early Child Development (ECD), and school health and nutrition. Efforts should be made to treat and prevent disease at the earliest opportunity to avoid substantial impairment to education. But these efforts should also continue in order to ensure that children are free of disease during the school-age years when they are learning and growing. We present evidence for the effects of health and nutrition on education from all stages of childhood before focusing on the programmatic advantages of delivering services to school-age children in the latter sections of the book.

A second conclusion from the review of evidence in Chapters 3, 4 and 5 is that **improving children's health and nutrition brings substantial benefits for cognitive development and education.** It is perhaps surprising that relatively short-term and simple health interventions can have substantial effects on children's learning. The evidence shows that improvements in cognitive skills and in educational achievement from health and nutrition interventions are substantial and match those due to more costly and intensive educational interventions.

As discussed above, the benefits of school health and nutrition interventions accrue disproportionately to the disadvantaged. In general, **improving health and nutrition brings the greatest educational benefits to the poor and most vulnerable.** In some cases, greater benefits are seen for children suffering from several conditions of ill health. For example, the greatest benefits of deworming are seen for children with heavy worm loads and who also have poor nutritional status. In many countries, girls' education is disadvantaged. Malaria prevention can help reduce the enrolment gap between girls and boys. Health and nutrition interventions also help the most economically disadvantaged. Early childhood nutritional supplements have a greater long-term effect for children from poor families. Thus, there are many ways in which improving health and nutrition brings the greatest educational benefits to the poor and most vulnerable.

A final conclusion from the review of evidence is that **health and education reinforce one another.** There are many examples in this book where a health programme and an education programme worked together to improve children's cognitive development or educational outcomes. There are examples where a combination of nutritional supplementation and an early childhood education programme was required to reverse cognitive delays of undernourished children. There are other examples where nutritional supplements in early childhood improve the effectiveness of a psychosocial programme to stimulate cognitive development. In school-age children, one example of a deworming programme did not benefit educational achievement of children but it did improve their ability to learn a new task that was taught to them. Education and health work together in many ways. Improving children's health at a time when they are learning maximises the possibility for this synergy.

Chapter 6 considers the costs and benefits of implementing school health and nutrition programmes. A major advancement in improving the health and nutrition of school-age children came with the development of programmes delivered through the education system. Training teachers to give treatments to children reduced the cost of delivering treatment for intestinal worms by a factor of 10. This means that **improving health and nutrition through schools can be highly cost-effective.** When health and nutrition interventions are delivered through the education system their cost-effectiveness compares favourably with other programmes to improve educational outcomes. For example, deworming interventions and conditional cash transfers both lead to an increase in the time children spend at school but deworming comes in at around one-fiftieth of the cost of cash transfer programmes per additional year of schooling. Chapter 6 goes on to estimate the likely global impact of school health and nutrition programmes considering that the diseases they treat are very prevalent and that they bring substantial benefits for education (discussed above). In this estimate, between 200 and 500 million years of schooling are lost to health and nutrition problems each year. Worm infections, undernutrition and anaemia are responsible for between 15 and 45 million additional cases of mental retardation. The global impact is enormous but so is the potential for school health and nutrition programmes to benefit children across the world. Our estimates suggest that **school health and nutrition interventions can have a massive global impact.**

In *Chapter 7*, policy options are considered for the implementation of such school health and nutrition programmes. A case is made for the public funding of these programmes because private financing cannot guarantee that services will reach the poorest. One of the major advantages of school health and nutrition programmes is that **programmes delivered through schools are sustainable and reach the poorest.** Alternatives (such as mobile health units) are rarely sustainable or cost-effective. Many ways of delivering treatments to children rely on proximity to urban centres, far from the marginalised rural poor. By contrast, most children attend schools. Services delivered through schools have a built-in mechanism to ensure sustainability and they reach the children who need them most.

We believe these arguments present a compelling case for school health and nutrition programmes. They are a "quick win", highly cost-effective, pro-poor, sustainable and they can have a massive global impact. The following pages will develop this overall argument in some detail. Evidence is reviewed comprehensively, allowing readers to assess the effectiveness of different interventions package of services. We hope to convince you that school health and nutrition programmes really are an urgent education policy priority for all poor countries.

Chapter 2

Challenges for child health and nutrition

In this chapter we ask: Which diseases affect children? Who is most susceptible to these diseases? How do threats from disease change with age throughout childhood? How can these diseases be effectively treated or prevented? We do not directly address education in this chapter but all the diseases we discuss – the most common conditions of poor health and nutrition in the world – affect children's education in one way or another, as detailed in Chapters 3, 4, and 5.

The opening chapter outlined the compelling case for school health and nutrition programmes and offered detailed arguments in support of this case. Four of these arguments related to the challenges facing child health and nutrition and are developed in this chapter. The first three of these relate to children of all ages: diseases that affect education are very prevalent; the poor are more likely to suffer from poor health and nutrition; diseases that affect education are preventable and treatable. These three themes run through both sections of this chapter looking first at the diseases of early childhood and then at diseases among school-age children. The fourth theme of this chapter relates specifically to children of school-age: schoolchildren bear the greatest burden of some of the most common diseases that affect education. The second half of this chapter looks at the changes in the disease profile affecting children throughout their childhood. We find that diseases such as worm infections become a more significant cause of illness for children as they reach school-age. At the same time, effective strategies exist for controlling such diseases among this population.

Health and nutrition of infants and preschool children

We begin with an analysis of the diseases affecting children before they reach school-age. Initially, child survival is the priority and we first look at the major

©CAB International 2008. *School Health, Nutrition and Education for All:* 11 *Levelling the Playing Field (*M.C.H. Jukes *et al.)*

causes of child mortality. As children increasingly survive such severe illnesses they face other challenges. Most of the diseases discussed in the following sections also affect children's development and subsequently their educational opportunities.

Out of 100 children born every year, 30 will most likely suffer from malnutrition in their first 5 years of life, 26 will not be immunised against the basic childhood diseases, 19 will lack access to safe drinking water, and 40 to adequate sanitation. In poor countries, every fourth child lives in abject poverty, in families with an income of less than US$1 a day. As a consequence nearly 11 million children each year – about 30,000 children a day – die before reaching their fifth birthday, mostly from preventable causes. Of these children, 4 million die in their first month of life. In many of the world's poorest countries, child mortality rates have either not changed or have worsened. In sub-Saharan Africa, child mortality averages 173 deaths per 1,000 live births, and in South Asia 98 deaths per 1,000 – many times the industrialised country average of 7 deaths per 1,000.

Treating health and nutrition problems in preschool children (under 5 years old) is important because of the prevalence of these problems and their association with poverty. That is, preschool children account for more than 50 per cent of the global gap in mortality between the poorest 20 per cent and richest 20 per cent of the world's population, and they bear 30 per cent of the total burden of disease in poor countries. Treating disease in this age group is therefore a very effective way to promote equity in health outcomes.

There are an estimated 600 million preschool children worldwide[1] and they have several-fold higher case fatality rates for many infections compared with other age groups; therefore keeping them healthy gives them a better chance of survival to adulthood. Of the 10.5 million children that died in 1999, 99 per cent were from poor countries and of these 36 per cent were in Asia and 33 per cent in Africa. Mortality results from infectious disease and a combination of other perinatal conditions, including malnutrition. The next section addresses these leading causes of mortality.

Health and nutrition in infancy and early childhood

More than 50 per cent of all deaths in children under 5 are due to five communicable diseases, which are treatable and preventable. These are pneumonia, diarrhoea, measles, malaria and HIV&AIDS (see Table 2.1 and Figure 2.1).

Pneumonia causes 2 million deaths annually

Pneumonia, or inflammation of the lung, is caused by a number of bacterial, fungal and viral infections[2]. Approximately 5 to 10 per cent of all children younger than 5 years old develop pneumonia each year and acute respiratory tract infections (ARTIs) cause approximately 2 million deaths each year among children under 5 years old, making them together one of the leading causes of death in this age group[3]. About 1 per cent of pneumonia cases have serious consequences (e.g. bronchiectasis), which increase the risk of recurrent infections. There has been some decrease in the number of pneumonia deaths over the last decade due to more widespread use of antibiotics; however the increasing prevalence of HIV infection in Africa has likely led to an increase in bacterial pneumonia there. Nearly 75 per cent of pneumonia deaths occur among infants under 12 months. The risk also increases with malnutrition, malaria and suppressed immunity. Treatment is with oral antibiotics in mild cases, or in more severe cases, hospitalisation and intravenous antibiotics.

Diarrhoea causes 21 per cent of deaths in children under 5 years

Diarrhoea is caused by several important bacterial and protozoal infections including *Vibrio cholerae, Escherichia coli* (0157), *Giardia lamblia, Cryptosporidium parvum* and *Entamoeba histolytica*. It is estimated to cause up to 2.5 million deaths a year in preschool children (21 per cent of total deaths of under 5 year olds)[4]. There has been a decline over the last 10 years, attributed to use of oral rehydration therapy, improved nutrition, immunisation and sanitation/hygiene. Treatment may be with oral rehydration therapy, which is, importantly, given as soon as possible; or with drugs aimed at the causative organism: antibiotics in the case of *V. cholerae* or *E. coli*, or antiprotozoals in the case of *G. lamblia, C. parvum* and *E. histolytica*. However, currently only around 30 per cent of under 5 year olds with diarrhoea use oral rehydration (see Table 2.3).

Malaria kills a child in Africa every 30 seconds

Malaria is a life threatening parasitic disease caused by *Plasmodium* spp. and transmitted by mosquitoes. It accounts for 1 in 5 of all childhood deaths in Africa. Anaemia, low birth weight, epilepsy, and neurological problems, all frequent consequences of malaria, compromise the health and development of millions of children throughout the tropical world. Malaria symptoms appear about 9 to 14 days after the infectious mosquito bite, although this varies with different *Plasmodium* species. Typically, malaria produces fever, headache, vomiting and other flu-like symptoms. If drugs are not available for treatment or the parasites are resistant to them, the infection can progress rapidly to become life threatening. Malaria can kill by infecting and destroying red blood cells (anaemia) and by clogging the capillaries that carry blood to the brain (cerebral malaria) or other vital organs. Treatment with antimalarials can be effective if

Table 2.1. Global burden of disease by DALYs and mortality. *Source:* WHO, World Health Report (2004)[5].

Disease	DALYs[*]	Mortality[**]
Measles	21463	611
Diarrhoeal disease	61926	1797
Pertussis	15587	293
Meningitis	5850	160
Malaria	46455	1272
Trypanosomiasis & Leishmaniasis	4274	114
Schistosomiasis	1696	16
Gastrointestinal helminths	2950	11
Otitis media	1432	3
Protein energy malnutrition	16893	260
Iodine deficiency	3518	5
Vitamin A deficiency	793	22
Iron deficiency anaemia	12209	137

[*]Estimated as one year lost of 'healthy' life, summed as years of life lost and years lost due to disability.

[**]Deaths per million of population.

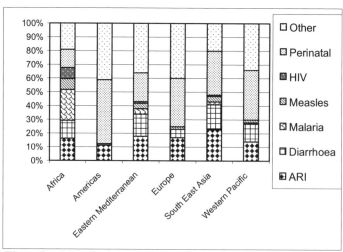

Figure 2.1. Mortality in under 5 year olds by disease and world region.

Table 2.2. Global nutrition indicators for early childhood.

| SUMMARY INDICATORS | % of infants with low birth weight 1998-2003 | % of children (1995-2003) who are: | | | % of under-fives (1995-2003) suffering from: | | | | Vitamin A supplementation coverage rate (6-59 months) 2002 | % of households consuming iodised salt 1997-2003 |
		exclusively breastfed (<6 months)	breastfed with complementary food (6-9 months)	Still breastfeeding (20-23 months)	underweight Moderate & severe	underweight severe	wasting Moderate & severe	stunting Moderate & severe		
Sub-Saharan Africa	14	28	64	51	29	8	9	38	71	67
Middle East and North Africa	15	32	59	25	14	2	6	21	-	57
South Asia	30	36	46	67	46	16	15	44	46	49
East Asia and Pacific	8	52	-	-	17	3	3	19	78e	84
Latin America and Caribbean	10	-	48	26	7	1	2	16	-	86
CEE/CIS	9	14	42	25	6	1	4	16	-	43
Industrialised countries	7	-	-	-	-	-	-	-	-	-
Developing countries	17	38	55	51	27	8	8	31	59	69
Least developed countries	18	33	63	63	36	10	10	42	70	52
World	16	37	55	51	27	8	8	31	-	67

e: This regional figure for East Asia and Pacific does not include China. *Source:* UNICEF (2005)[6].

delivered quickly after the onset of a fever. However, because of the rise of drug resistance in many areas, the most successful treatment regime recommended by WHO is with combination therapy, preferably with artemisinin-based combination therapy (ACT)[7]. It is vital in the treatment of malaria to provide rapid diagnosis and prompt treatment, but these are proving to be the greatest challenges in malaria prevention.

Today approximately 40 per cent of the world's population, mostly those living in the world's poorest countries, are at risk of malaria. It is found throughout the tropical and sub-tropical regions of the world and causes more than 300 million acute episodes and at least 1 million deaths annually, 90 per cent of which occur in sub-Saharan Africa among young children. Malaria kills an African child every 30 seconds. Many children who survive an episode of severe malaria suffer from learning impairments or brain damage (discussed in Chapter 4). Pregnant women and their unborn children are also particularly vulnerable to malaria, which is a major cause of perinatal mortality, low birth weight and maternal anaemia. In sub-Saharan Africa 14 per cent of children under 5 sleep under a bednet, 2 per cent sleep under a bednet treated with insecticide and 38 per cent of those with fever receive antimalarial drugs (see Table 2.3).

Measles results in more than 700,000 child deaths annually

Forty years after effective vaccines were licensed, measles continues to cause death and severe disease in children worldwide. Measles is caused by the measles virus and its main symptoms are a running nose, cough, conjunctivitis and high fever, leading to the appearance of a skin rash. Complications from measles can occur in almost every organ system. Pneumonia, croup and encephalitis are common causes of death; encephalitis is the most common cause of long-term impairment. Measles remains a common cause of blindness in poor countries. Complication rates are higher in those under 5 and over 20 years old, although croup and otitis media are more common in those under 2 years old and encephalitis in older children and adults. Complication rates are increased by immune deficiency disorders, malnutrition, vitamin A deficiency, intense exposures to measles, and lack of previous measles vaccination. Case fatality rates have decreased with improvements in socioeconomic status in many countries but remain high in poor countries. In 2000, the World Health Organisation estimated that between 30 and 40 million persons developed measles, resulting in 777,000 child deaths, most in sub-Saharan Africa. High case fatality rates in poor countries are a result from infection at a young age, crowding, underlying immune deficiency disorders, vitamin A deficiency, and lack of access to medical care. An estimated 125 million preschool-age children are thought to have vitamin A deficiency, placing them at high risk for death, severe infection, or blindness as a result of measles, because vitamin A is important for the strength of the skin and membranes of the eye, respiratory tree and gut[8]. In poor countries, measles case fatality rates are 10 to 100 fold higher than in rich countries. Ten per cent of infections develop serious, severe complications[9]. While there is no specific treatment for measles infection, prevention is by vaccination; treating the secondary (bacterial) infections and fever in infected children is recommended, as well as vitamin A supplementation, to reduce the incidence of measles-associated deaths in the developing world. Eradication of measles by vaccination would be a major public health accomplishment. To prevent epidemics occurring 85 per cent of children must become immune to the disease. This is equivalent to 98 per cent coverage rate of immunisation. Currently only 67 per cent of infants are immunised against measles in least developed countries (Table 2.3).

More than 1,500 children are infected with HIV every day

Every day more than 1,500 children become infected with HIV[10]. Children may acquire HIV from their mother during pregnancy, labour, delivery or breast-feeding, with estimates of mother-to-child transmission (MTCT) at between 15 and 25 per cent without the use of antiretroviral drugs. Other routes of infection are through blood transfusion, the use of contaminated syringes and needles, and child sex abuse[11]. Children with HIV infection suffer the same common childhood diseases as other children, but more frequently, with greater intensity and often with a poorer response to drugs. Illnesses that are rarely fatal in healthy children will cause high mortality in the HIV-infected child. Without access to antiretroviral therapy, disease progression is rapid and 45 per cent of infected children will die before the age of 2[10]. Prevention of MTCT is best effected by preventing infection in women or preventing unintentional pregnancies in HIV-positive women or by treating the mother with antiretroviral therapy during pregnancy, birth and administered to the baby after birth. To reduce the impact of HIV infection on children, early diagnosis is required and the child should receive good nutrition and appropriate immunisations and drug therapy for treating common childhood infections[10].

Malnutrition and other perinatal conditions cause 20 per cent of child deaths

Perinatal conditions account for more than 1 in 5 deaths among children under 5. Most deaths are the result of poor maternal health and nutrition, inadequate care during pregnancy and delivery, lack of essential care for the newborn baby, infections, birth injury, asphyxia and problems relating to premature births. Malnutrition influences the effect of these conditions. Childhood underweight is an important public health problem and its devastating effects on human performance, health and survival are well established. It is estimated that about

Table 2.3. Global health indicators for early childhood.

SUMMARY INDICATORS	% of population using improved drinking water sources 2002			% of population using adequate sanitation facilities 2002			% of routine EPI vaccines financed by government 2003	% immunised 2003 1-year-old children				
	total	urban	rural	total	urban	rural	total	TB	DPT3	polio	measles	hepB 3
Sub-Saharan Africa	57	82	44	36	55	26	45	74	60	63	62	30
Middle East and North Africa	87	95	77	72	88	52	89	88	87	87	88	71
South Asia	84	94	80	35	64	23	96	82	71	72	67	1
East Asia and Pacific	78	92	68	50	72	35	84	91	86	87	82	66
Latin America and Caribbean	89	95	69	75	84	44	92	96	89	91	93	73
CEE/CIS	91	98	79	81	92	62	89	95	88	89	90	81
Industrialised countries	100	100	100	100	100	100	69	-	95	93	92	62
Developing countries	79	92	70	49	73	31	80	85	76	77	75	40
Least developed countries	58	80	50	35	58	27	37	79	68	68	67	20
World	83	95	72	58	81	37	80	85	78	79	77	42

Table 2.3. *continued.* Global health indicators for early childhood.

SUMMARY INDICATORS	% immunised 2003 — pregnant women tetanus	% under-fives with ARI (1998-2003)	% under-fives with ARI taken to health provider (1998-2003)	% under-fives with diarrhoea receiving oral rehydration and continued feeding 1994-2003	Malaria: 1999-2003 — % under-fives sleeping under a bednet	Malaria: 1999-2003 — % under-fives sleeping under a treated bednet	Malaria: 1999-2003 — % under-fives with fever receiving anti-malarial drugs
Sub-Saharan Africa	53	14	39	32	14	2	38
Middle East and North Africa	-	12	69	-	-	-	-
South Asia	75	19	57	26	-	-	-
East Asia and Pacific	-	-	-	-	-	-	-
Latin America and Caribbean	-	-	-	36	-	-	-
CEE/CIS	-	-	-	25	-	-	-
Industrialised countries	-	-	-	-	-	-	-
Developing countries	64	16	52	31	-	-	-
Least developed countries	56	16	37	35	19	2	36
World	64	16	53	31	-	-	-

Source: UNICEF (2005)[6].

53 per cent of all deaths in young children are contributed to underweight, varying from 45 per cent for deaths due to measles to 61 per cent for deaths due to diarrhoea. The vast majority of underweight children live in poorer regions, mainly in Asia and Africa. The projected trends in the prevalence of underweight children combined with the different population growth these regions are experiencing (increasing in Africa, decreasing in Asia) will narrow the gap between their respective contributions to the total number of underweight children. While in 1990, of 100 underweight children, 80 were estimated to live in Asia and 16 in Africa; in 2015, these numbers are expected to change to 60 and 38, respectively, if recent trends continue[12]. Recent statistics[6,13] indicate that the prevalence of moderate and severe stunting in under 5 year olds is 42 per cent in least developed countries (44 per cent in South Asia and 38 per cent in sub-Saharan Africa; Table 2.2). This figure has reduced from 47 per cent (52 per cent in South Asia and 41 per cent in sub-Saharan Africa) since 1998. Prevalence of moderate and severe underweight has fallen to 36 per cent (46 per cent in South Asia, 29 per cent in sub-Saharan Africa; Table 2.2) from 40 per cent (51 per cent in South Asia, 32 per cent in sub-Saharan Africa) since 1998.

Low birth weight is another common form of malnutrition, also with severe consequences. The majority of low birth weight in developing countries is due to low *in utero* growth rates, influenced by maternal undernutrition, malaria, anaemia and chronic/acute infections, such as sexually transmitted infections (STIs) and urinary tract infections (UTIs). Consequences of low birth weight are impaired immune function, poor cognitive development for neonates and infants, increased risk of diarrhoeal diseases and pneumonia/lower respiratory tract infections (LRTIs).

Micronutrient deficiencies in children are less apparent than underweight and stunting but represent some of the most common forms of malnutrition worldwide, with consequences for physical and mental development. The most common is iron deficiency, with a worldwide prevalence of 2 billion. Forty to fifty per cent of under 5 year olds in developing countries are thought to be iron deficient[14]. Implications for mental development are discussed in Chapters 4 and 5.

Diseases of early childhood are preventable and treatable

All of the childhood diseases discussed in this section are preventable or treatable. Diarrhoea can be prevented through improved health and sanitation and can be treated with oral rehydration salts. Pneumonia can be treated with antibiotics. Malaria can be prevented with insecticide treated bednets and can be treated with antimalarial drugs. There is a vaccine for measles. Mother-to-child transmission from HIV can be virtually eliminated through the use of antiretroviral treatment. Nutritional supplementation and improved diet can prevent and treat malnutrition. Given that these diseases are highly prevalent and are concentrated among the poorest communities, this amounts to a massive avoidable loss of life and potential in poor countries. The loss of educational potential is the focus of this book and the following chapters consider the long-term effects of disease in early childhood on education access and achievement. The educational impact of poor health and nutrition is probably more apparent when considering the diseases affecting school-age children. It is to these diseases that we turn next.

Summary: Health and nutrition in infancy and early childhood

- More than 50 per cent of all child deaths (under 5 years old) are due to five communicable diseases. These are pneumonia, diarrhoea, measles, malaria and HIV&AIDS.
- Five to ten per cent of under 5 year olds develop pneumonia each year, with 2 million deaths overall due to acute respiratory tract infections.
- Two and a half million deaths are due to diarrhoea, accounting for 21 per cent of all deaths in under 5 year olds. Only 30 per cent of this age group use oral rehydration to treat diarrhoea.
- Malaria causes 300 million acute episodes and 1 million deaths, mostly in under 5 year olds. In sub-Saharan Africa, only 2 per cent of this age group sleep under an insecticide-treated bednet.
- Around 800,000 childhood deaths are caused by measles, a figure which is increased by the high prevalence of vitamin A deficiency among preschool children, at 125 million worldwide. Sixty-seven per cent of children under 12 months receive measles vaccinations in least developed countries.
- Mortality due to all these diseases is increased by HIV infection. Fifteen hundred children become infected with HIV everyday. Forty-five per cent of these will die before age 2 without access to antiretroviral therapy.
- Malnutrition and other perinatal conditions account for 20 per cent of childhood deaths. Underweight is estimated to contribute to 53 per cent of all childhood deaths. The prevalences of moderate to severe stunting and underweight are 42 per cent and 36 per cent respectively. Both figures have fallen by around 5 per cent since 1998. Forty to fifty per cent of under 5 year olds are iron deficient, with implications for their development.
- All these leading causes of childhood illness are either preventable or treatable.

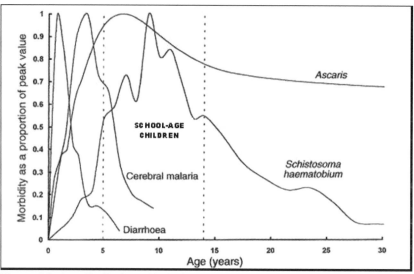

Figure 2.2. Age distribution of infection-specific mortality. *Source:* Bundy & Guyatt (1996)[15].

School-age children

Due to the success of child survival programmes, there is an ever increasing number of children reaching school-age (defined here as 5 to 14 years). There are an estimated 1,200 million children of school-age worldwide, with 88 per cent of these living in poorer countries[1]. However, a growing awareness and understanding of the heavy burden of disease and malnutrition among school-age children has prompted increasing concern as to the negative consequences of these insults on a child's long-term development[16,17]. As much of the burden derives from poverty-related issues, it is the 88 per cent of children living in poorer countries who are most at risk.

Disease

Children harbour greater worm loads as they reach school-age

As Figure 2.2 demonstrates, the diseases most important to the preschool child, for example, cerebral malaria and diarrhoea-related illness, become less important to the school-age child, as other diseases become more important, for example, infections with parasitic worms (such as roundworm, whipworm, hookworm and the schistosomes), also known as helminths. It is estimated that between 25 and 35 per cent of school-age children are infected with one or more of the major helminth species[18-20].

The prevalence of helminth infections rises to a maximum in childhood and settles to a stable plateau in the adult population (see Figure 2.3). However, as demonstrated in Figure 2.4, there is a marked peak in the age-intensity profile. This shows that it is the school-age child that harbours the most intense infections. Because morbidity is directly related to the intensity of infection, it follows that it is this age group who carry the greatest burden of disease[21]. The intestinal worms, *Ascaris lumbricoides* (roundworm) and *Trichuris trichiura* (whipworm) account for an estimated 12 per cent and 11 per cent respectively of the total disease burden for this age group, making this group of worm infections the single largest contributor to the disease burden of this group. An estimated 20 per cent of disability adjusted life years (DALYs) lost due to communicable disease among schoolchildren are a direct result of infection with intestinal helminths[22].

As numbers of worms harboured in the infected child build up over time, many of the health problems are chronic and can be long-lasting. In addition, polyparasitism is a common occurrence: children may be concurrently infected with several parasite species[23]. Children with chronic worm infections may be stunted and underweight, which can lead to long-term retardation of mental and physical development, even death in severe cases. Infection can also contribute to malnutrition through lack of appetite, malabsorption and anaemia through loss of blood. The intestinal worms (*Ascaris lumbricoides*, *Trichuris trichiura* and the hookworms *Necator americanus* and *Ancylostoma duodenale*) are easily treated with a single dose of albendazole and mebendazole once a year or more (in areas with less than 50 per cent prevalence). This cheap, readily available and

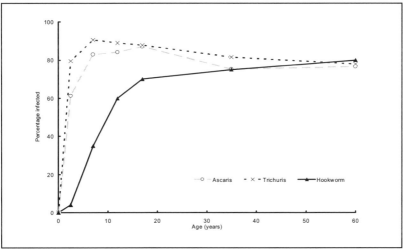

Figure 2.3. Prevalence of helminth infection, by age. *Source:* Bundy et al. (1992)[24].

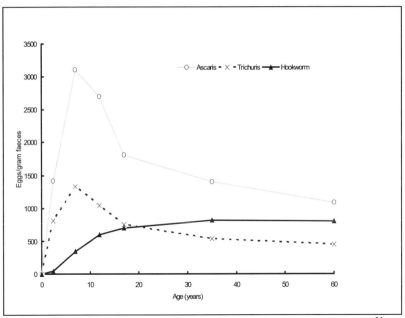

Figure 2.4. Intensity of helminth infection, by age. *Source:* Bundy *et al.* (1992)[24].

easily tolerated treatment can be administered through schools by teachers for greater cost benefit[23]. Intestinal and urinary bilharzia or schistosomiasis, caused by the blood flukes *Schistosoma mansoni* and *S. haematobium* are also treated easily with a single dose of praziquantel, which can also be delivered through the school system[23].

Malaria continues to affect children in school-age

Some diseases are of greater importance to the preschool child, but still reflect a significant burden of disease for the school-age child. A good example of this is malaria. In areas of unstable transmission, a child will suffer fewer episodes, resulting in a slower build up of exposure-driven immunity and a greater risk of severe and fatal consequences in children[25,26]. Recent preliminary estimates suggest that malaria accounts for 10 to 20 per cent of all-cause mortality among school-age children[27].

Malaria is also an important cause of morbidity, but this does appear to decline rapidly with age: children aged 5 to 9 years experience between 0.25 and 2.3 malaria attacks per annum, whereas children aged 10 to 20 years experience between only 0.1 and 1.3 attacks per annum[28]. Nevertheless, malaria remains a major cause of absenteeism and cognitive impairment in school-age children (discussed in Chapters 3 and 4).

HIV&AIDS leaves millions of school-age children without parents

HIV infection prevalence is lowest in the age group 5 to 14 years (see Figure 2.5). However, there are an estimated 3.8 million children under the age of 15 who have been infected with HIV since the epidemic began. More than two-thirds have since died, the vast majority of these from sub-Saharan Africa[10].

The relatively low prevalence of HIV&AIDS in school-age children means that the direct effects of AIDS-related illness constitute a relatively small proportion of the total burden of disease. In contrast, the indirect effects are enormous. Children may suffer physically, socially and psychologically through a death or illness of a family member – most likely their parents[11, 29-31].

One of the greatest impacts is the number of children orphaned by this pandemic. Orphans are among the most vulnerable people in society. The proportion of orphans has risen from 2 per cent to almost 15 per cent in some African countries, with AIDS accounting for 50 per cent of this increase[32]. This translates into over 13 million children under the age of 15, having lost either their mother or both parents to AIDS. In less than 10 years time, the figure is expected to reach more than 25 million[11, 29].

However, the school-age child does offer a "window of hope" for the next generation. There is no cure for HIV&AIDS, but prevention methods are effective and the spread of the disease is by no means inevitable. Schools have the opportunity to reach large numbers of children and young people delivering the "social vaccine" of education, helping them to adopt healthy ways of behaving and to protect themselves from infection[29].

Malnutrition

Stunting and underweight increase throughout the school-age years

Stunting (low height-for-age) is a physical indicator of chronic or long-term undernutrition (lack of calories or protein) and is often linked to poor mental development. It is widely believed to occur mainly in early childhood (mostly by 3 years of age) and through a cumulative process of poor growth. Children stunted at school-age are likely to have been exposed to poor nutrition since early childhood. Underweight (low weight-for-age) is an indicator of both chronic and acute undernutrition and is also common in school-age children.

A large study of the heights and weights of rural schoolchildren in a number of low income countries found the overall prevalence of both stunting and underweight to be high, ranging from 48 to 56 per cent for stunting and 34 to 62 per cent for underweight[33]. It has also been noted that children become progressively shorter with age, relative to the reference population (see Figure 2.6), and that boys are more stunted than girls.

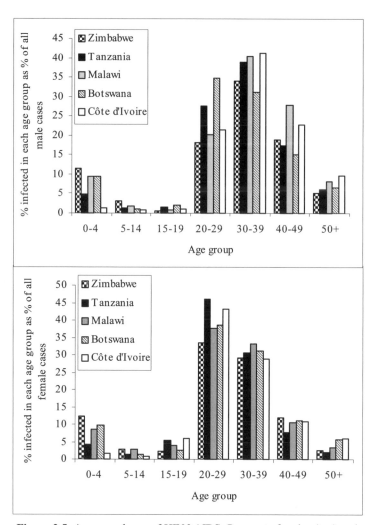

Figure 2.5. Age prevalence of HIV&AIDS. Per cent of males (top) and females (bottom) infected with HIV in each age group (as a percentage of all HIV infected males and females, respectively), for five countries in Africa. Infection peaks at a younger age in women than in men. *Source:* UNAIDS epidemiological fact sheets, 2000[34].

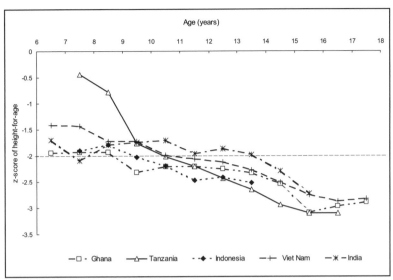

Figure 2.6. Mean z-scores of height-for-age of boys in five countries (z-scores of <-2 indicate stunting). *Source:* Partnership for Child Development (1998)[33].

Anaemia affects 40 per cent of African schoolchildren

In addition to a lack of protein or calories in children's diet, there may also be a lack of small quantities of essential vitamins and minerals, known as micronutrients. Nutritional anaemia, particularly deficiencies of iron, iodine and vitamin A are major problems for school-age children, with multiple micronutrient deficiencies being a common occurrence. It has been shown that such deficiencies can negatively impact on growth, increase susceptibility to infection and also impair mental development and learning ability.

Iron deficiency is the most common of these disorders and can be caused by insufficient intake of iron-rich foods, parasitic infections (particularly hookworm and malaria) and deficiencies of other nutrients[35-37]. It is estimated that 53 per cent of school-age children suffer from iron deficiency anaemia[38]. In a survey of nearly 14,000 rural schoolchildren in Africa and Asia, prevalence of anaemia was more than 40 per cent in the African countries surveyed and between 12 and 28 per cent in Asia (see Figure 2.7)[39]. In areas where malaria is endemic, the disease may be the primary cause of half of all severe cases of anaemia. For children, health consequences include premature birth, low birth weight, infections and elevated risk of death. Physical and cognitive developments are also impaired, resulting in poorer school performance (discussed in Chapter 5).

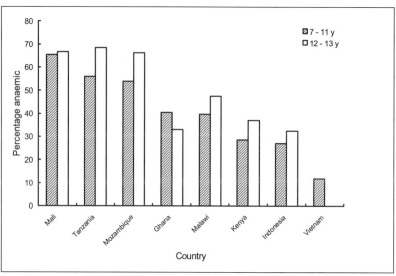

Figure 2.7. Prevalence of anaemia in school-age children in eight countries in Africa and Asia. *Source*: Partnership for Child Development (2001)[39].

Iodine deficiency is the leading preventable cause of mental retardation

Iodine deficiency disorders (IDD) affect an estimated 60 million (5 per cent) school-age children. Serious iodine deficiency during pregnancy may result in stillbirths and abortions. Such deficiency may also result in congenital abnormalities such as cretinism, a grave, irreversible form of mental retardation that affects people living in iodine deficient areas of Africa and Asia. Older children living in these areas may continue to suffer ill health and poor cognitive development. Recent studies of schoolchildren in Egypt, Swaziland and South Africa have found prevalence rates of 35 to 70 per cent, indicating a severe public health problem in the school-age population[40-42]. IDD affects poor, pregnant women and preschool children, posing serious public health problems in 130 poor countries. Nearly 50 million people suffer from some degree of IDD-related brain damage.

Vitamin A deficiency affects 85 million school-age children

Vitamin A deficiency affects an estimated 85 million (7 per cent) school-age children. The deficiency causes impaired immune function and iron metabolism, and confers an increased risk of mortality from infectious disease and is widely recognised as an important cause of blindness in children. The small number of

Summary: School-age children

- 25 to 35 per cent of school-age children are infected with one or more of the major helminth species. An estimated 20 per cent of disability adjusted life years (DALYs) lost due to communicable disease among schoolchildren are a direct result of intestinal helminths. Single dose treatments are available for all major species of helminth.
- Malaria is a less significant problem for children once they reach school-age but it is still responsible for 10 to 20 per cent of all-cause mortality in this age group.
- 13 million children under the age of 15 have lost either their mother or both parents to AIDS. In less than 10 years' time, the figure is expected to reach more than 25 million.
- 48 to 56 per cent of school-age children are stunted and 34 to 62 per cent are underweight.
- 53 per cent of school-age children suffer from iron deficiency anaemia.
- Iodine deficiency disorders affect an estimated 60 million (5 per cent) school-aged children. Vitamin A deficiency affects an estimated 85 million (7 per cent).

recent studies conducted, suggest that this is also a major public health problem in school-age children[43]. Vitamin A deficiency is a public health problem in 118 countries, especially in Africa and South-East Asia, once again hitting hardest young children and pregnant women in low income countries. Between 100 and 140 million children are vitamin A deficient. An estimated 250,000 to 500,000 vitamin A deficient children become blind every year, half of them dying within 12 months of losing their sight[44]. Supplementing vitamin A between 6 months and 6 years of age can reduce overall child mortality by a quarter in areas with significant vitamin A deficiency. However, because breast-feeding is time-limited and the effects of vitamin A supplementation capsules last only 4 to 6 months, neither are long-term solutions. Rather, they should be seen as initial steps towards better overall nutrition[44].

Increasing numbers of schoolchildren are overweight

There are an estimated 17.6 million children who are overweight. This condition begins in preschool children and becomes more evident among school-age children[45]. In sub-Saharan Africa and Asia, this is still a rare condition, but in the richer countries of Latin America, the Middle East, Central Europe and North Africa, overweight and obesity are as common as in the United States. Countries undergoing the "nutrition transition" also have high levels of stunting which is believed to be a risk factor for obesity. It is suggested that the increased risk of obesity among stunted children will lead to considerable problems with obesity in children in low income countries in the coming decades.

Conclusion

The diseases discussed in this chapter illustrate four reasons why health and nutrition programmes are so important.

Diseases that affect education are very prevalent

The numbers are staggering. Half of all schoolchildren have anaemia. Half of them are stunted in growth as a result of undernutrition. One-third have worm infections. Any effect these diseases have on education will be multiplied by hundreds of millions of children who suffer these conditions of poor health and nutrition. The cumulative worldwide loss of intellectual potential is enormous.

The poor are more likely to suffer from poor health and nutrition

Children in rich communities do not contract HIV from their mothers. Few of them die of measles, have worm infections or are stunted in growth. The poor bear the burden of the world's diseases. Children in poor communities lack educational opportunities for many reasons and poor health and nutrition are just additional barriers between them and their educational potential. But tackling children's health and nutrition is one way to reduce inequalities in education. This is because most of these diseases are preventable and treatable.

Diseases that affect education are preventable and treatable

All of the major diseases affecting education are preventable and treatable, whether through vaccines, pills, improved hygiene or behaviour change. The lost educational potential due to these diseases is entirely avoidable.

Schoolchildren bear the greatest burden of some of the most common diseases that affect education

Strategies to control disease among schoolchildren are particularly effective. Deworming children every 6 months or so can prevent the illness that accompanies worm infections. Regular iron supplementation can help reduce the prevalence of anaemia. As the majority of worm infections and many cases of anaemia are concentrated in the school-age population, treating these children is an effective way to reduce the global impact of these diseases. This is part of what makes health and nutrition programmes targeted at school-age children such an attractive option.

We have presented the case for health and nutrition programmes arising from an understanding of the prevalence and distribution of disease throughout the world and the methods required to control these diseases. In the following three chapters we will consider the effects of these diseases on children's education. The next steps in our argument are to show that these prevalent and preventable diseases have a large impact on children's education. The impact is felt from the diseases in infancy and early childhood through to those affecting children when they are attending primary school. We will consider these effects throughout childhood before focusing, in the latter sections of the book, at programmes specific to school-age children. We begin, in Chapter 3, by looking at the effects of poor health and nutrition on access to education.

Chapter 3

Health, nutrition and access to education

In the previous chapter we presented an analysis of the current challenges for children's health and nutrition and developed much of the rationale for health and nutrition programmes. Four of the arguments for health and nutrition programmes emerged: diseases that affect education are very prevalent; the poor are more likely to suffer from poor health and nutrition; all of these diseases are preventable and treatable; and schoolchildren bear the greatest burden of some of the most common diseases that affect education.

The next three chapters consider the impact of these diseases on education. In the current chapter we look at the impact of health and nutrition on access to education before going on, in Chapters 4 and 5, to examine the impact on children's learning once they do attend school.

Two further reasons to promote health and nutrition programmes emerge in the current chapter: disease affects education throughout childhood; health and nutrition interventions bring substantial benefits for education. Both of these arguments apply equally to learning outcomes, but we consider them first in the context of access to education.

Access to education is affected by health and nutrition throughout childhood because of the many different diseases that affect enrolment and attendance and because of the many mechanisms by which this effect occurs. Many children fail to enrol in school because of severe mental and physical disability resulting from poor health and nutrition. Less severe conditions also have consequences for access. Malaria and undernutrition both affect enrolment and drop-out. These two diseases, together with iron deficiency anaemia and worm infections also cause children to be absent from school. In many of these examples the effect of education is substantial. We will see how malaria in early childhood can lead to children dropping out of school a year prematurely; and how children with heavy

 ©CAB International 2008. *School Health, Nutrition and Education for All: Levelling the Playing Field (*M.C.H. Jukes *et al.)*

worm infections are absent from school for 30 per cent of the year – double the absenteeism rate for uninfected peers.

This chapter looks at these cases in detail in two sections. The first section considers the impact of health and nutrition on school enrolment, beginning with the diseases that have severe consequences and occur early in life and working up to the health of children at the age of enrolment. The second section looks at the impact on absenteeism and drop-out from preschools and primary schools. First, let us look at the current state of educational access in poor countries.

School enrolment, absenteeism and drop-out in poor countries

The initial challenge of universal primary education is getting children into school and keeping them there. Currently, 77 million children worldwide are out of school[1] and 33 countries are projected to miss the target of universal primary enrolment by 2015[2]. School completion is as much a problem as enrolment. For example, Malawi is a country which has made great progress towards educational access for all, with over 100 per cent gross enrolment ratio[a]. However, only 38 per cent of enrolled Malawian children complete basic education (4 years of primary schooling). According to current projections 80 countries are due to fail in their efforts to deliver basic education to all children by 2015. The situation is worse for girls. They are less likely than boys to enrol in school and less likely to complete their schooling once they have enrolled. Around one-third of all countries failed to achieve the target set for gender parity in primary education by 2005.

School absenteeism is common and also undermines educational efforts. Clearly, children who attend school less frequently are less likely to fulfil their educational potential. Chronic absenteeism can have most serious effects when it leads to grade repetition or drop-out from school.

Obstacles to educational access include the direct costs of sending children to school, requirement for children to work and the perception of the value of education and of school quality. However, as we shall see in this chapter, the health and nutrition of children also has a major role to play in achieving universal access to education. We look first at the impact on school enrolment.

---

[a] The gross enrolment ratio (GER) is the number of children attending primary schooling expressed as a percentage of the total school-age population. GERs >100 per cent are possible where children older than school-age are still attending primary school.

Health, nutrition and school enrolment

The health of children in the preschool years can affect the likelihood of their entering school for a number of reasons. For example, parents may choose not to invest in the education of a sickly child. Where illness has moderate effects on children's mental or physical abilities, parents may perceive them as less able than their siblings and less likely to benefit from schooling. But one of the most apparent ways in which children's chances of enrolling in school are affected by ill health is where disease leads to serious physical or mental disabilities. Such conditions typically affect children's educational opportunities to a greater extent in low income countries than in high income countries. This is not only because poorly resourced schools lack the facilities to cater for the special needs of children with disabilities but also because of the stigma that can be attached to these children, either from parents who do not think the child's education is worth investing in, or from fellow schoolchildren and teachers who do not wish to have them in their schools[3].

Surveys of the prevalence of disabilities in low income countries are relatively rare but sufficient data exist to suggest that a significant proportion of children are affected. For example, studies have found prevalence of serious mental retardation ranging from 5 children per 1,000 in Bangladesh, to 17 per 1,000 in Jamaica, 19 per 1,000 in Pakistan[4] and a study in South Africa[5] found around 35 children per 1,000 had intellectual disabilities. In the following sections, we consider the diseases of early childhood that can influence a child's chances of enrolling in school, either by causing severe physical or mental retardation or through more subtle effects that affect parental decisions about their children's schooling. We look first at diseases of poor nutrition and then at infectious diseases.

The impact of nutrition on primary school enrolment

Iodine and folate deficiencies can lead to severe mental and physical disability

Although few detailed data are available concerning the causes of disability in low income countries, it is clear that micronutrient deficiencies and their interactions with infections play a major role. The World Health Organisation estimates that vitamin A deficiency causes around 350,000 (~70 per cent) of new cases of blindness or partial blindness occurring in children each year. In addition to the direct effects of vitamin A deficiency on vision, it also contributes to childhood disability by increasing the risk of measles and other serious childhood infections that can result in long-term disability.

Iodine deficiency is still prevalent in many low income countries and is the leading cause of preventable mental retardation, worldwide. *In utero* exposure to maternal iodine deficiency during the first two trimesters of pregnancy can damage the developing brain, causing permanent cognitive disability as well as motor, hearing and speech disabilities[6]. Such iodine deficiency disorders can be totally eliminated by preventive measures using iodine administered in salt, oil or some other vehicle. In 1996, WHO reported that 56 per cent of the population of 83 poor countries now had adequate access to iodised salt. This represents an increase of 750 million people since 1990 with protection of 12 million children[7].

Folate deficiency very early in pregnancy can lead to neural tube defects, such as spina bifida, which results in motor disability and in some cases intellectual impairment in offspring. Data from South Africa put the prevalence of neural tube defects at between 0.63 and 1.74 per 1,000 live births, with higher prevalence for whites of European descent compared to black Africans[8]. More than half the cases of neural tube deficits can be prevented by giving supplementation of 400 micrograms (µg) of folic acid per day to women of childbearing age around the time of conception[9]. Thus, for all micronutrient deficiencies considered in this section, steps can be taken to prevent the impact on children's education potential.

Early childhood stunting has long-term effects on primary school enrolment

Stunting results from chronic undernutrition. Consequently, poor nutrition in early childhood may become most apparent later in life, in terms of the cumulative effects on a child's growth. Later on in this chapter we will see that children who are stunted at school-age are less likely to enrol on time and (in Chapter 5) that their achievement is also affected. There is also independent evidence of the effect of early childhood stunting on children's educational outcomes. The focus for many of these studies has been on assessing children's educational achievement and cognitive function, and these are discussed in Chapter 4. One study in the Philippines[10] also looked at children's enrolment, grade repetition and school attendance. The study found that children who were severely stunted before age 2 were more likely to enrol in school late, to repeat a grade, and to be absent from school. For many children undernutrition is ever present and its effects on education are felt at every point in the life cycle.

The impact of infection on primary school enrolment

Infection before birth can lead to disability

There are several infectious diseases which can lead to disabilities at birth. Maternal rubella infection in the early stages of pregnancy is highly likely to be transmitted to the infant and can lead to congenital rubella syndrome (CRS), the symptoms of which include deafness, cataracts, visual impairments, mental retardation and heart defects. Estimates[11] suggest that 110,000 cases of CRS occur every year in poor countries. Rubella can be controlled effectively through vaccination. Currently (in 2001) less than a third of low income countries included rubella in their national immunisation programmes, with virtually no countries in sub-Saharan Africa or South Asia systematically vaccinating against rubella. However, in countries with high transmission rates, immunity is also high and large-scale vaccination programmes may not necessarily be the best response.

Congenital syphilis can cause deafness and mental retardation in infected children. It is estimated that around 10 per cent of pregnant woman in many parts of sub-Saharan Africa are infected with syphilis[12] with around 12 million new infections each year[13], although rising levels of HIV infection are likely to result in an increase in the prevalence of syphilis. There are well established procedures of antenatal screening and treatment with penicillin[14] for the prevention of congenital syphilis but coverage is currently poor. So, the two most common forms of prenatal infection causing disability – syphilis and rubella – are straightforward to treat. The loss to education caused by these diseases is entirely avoidable. This applies equally to infectious diseases of early childhood, such as malaria, polio and meningitis, which we consider in the following sections.

Early childhood malaria prevention increases school enrolment

The most common infectious disease causing mental disability in low income countries is malaria. In its most extreme form, malaria attacks the brain (cerebral malaria) and can lead to neurological damage or death. In sub-Saharan Africa, cerebral malaria annually affects 575,000 children under 5 years of age, of whom 110,000 die. The survivors suffer developmental and behavioural impairments: each year, between 9,000 and 19,000 children (more than 2 per cent of survivors) less than 5 years of age in Africa, experience neurological complications lasting for more than 6 months[15]. These include hemiplegic cerebral palsy (involving paralysis of one side of the body), cortical blindness, motor coordination problems (ataxia) and language problems (aphasia)[16]. Such complications affect children's chances of going to school. A study in Kenya found that children who had suffered severe episodes of malaria with a high risk of neurological damage were less likely to have been enrolled in school than children with low levels of malaria infection[17]. One explanation for this is that parents recognise the cognitive delays suffered by their children and accordingly delay or abandon plans for their school enrolment.

Clear evidence of the impact of early childhood malaria on educational access comes from recent work in the Gambia[18]. In this study, children aged 6 months to 5 years, were given antimalarial drugs during consecutive malaria transmission seasons to protect them from malaria infection. The children were then followed for 15 years. This study found that prevention of early childhood malaria through regular chemoprophylaxis led to children staying at school for around one additional year (discussed in Chapter 4). The results also suggested a differential impact on school enrolment by gender, although with borderline statistical significance. In the early 1990s, when children in the study were attending school, gender differences in school enrolment in the Gambia were substantial. In this study, girls were six times less likely to be enrolled in school than boys. However, prevention of malaria doubled girls' chances of school enrolment and helped to reduce the gender gap in enrolment. This is one of the clearest examples of how improving children's health in the preschool years can lead to increased participation in primary schooling.

Polio infection causes severe disability

Other childhood diseases cause mental and physical disabilities which are likely to affect chances of school enrolment in resource-poor settings. Polio is a highly infectious disease caused by a virus which invades the nervous system and causes irreversible paralysis (usually of the legs) in around 1 in 200 cases. Children under 5 are most vulnerable to infection. Polio can be effectively controlled by use of an oral vaccine. The Global Polio Eradication Initiative has been successful with an estimated number of cases reduced from 350,000 at its launch in 1988 to fewer than 500 cases in 2001.

Meningitis leads to severe cognitive impairment

Another disease that directly affects the developing brain is meningitis, an inflammation of the lining around the brain and spinal cord caused by a number of different types of infections, but two types are predominant: pneumococcal meningitis and *Haemophilus influenzae* type b (Hib) meningitis. The disease often occurs in epidemics and is most prevalent in the "meningitis belt", an area extending across Africa from Ethiopia to Senegal. Globally, there are around 500,000 cases of meningitis each year, with very young children being at the greatest risk. Overall, around 10 per cent of cases are fatal and between 10 and 15 per cent of survivors suffer persistent neurological defects including hearing loss, speech disorders, mental retardation, seizures and motor impairment. However problems may be more severe in poor countries. A study in the Gambia found that death occurred in 48 per cent of children with pneumococcal meningitis and 58 per cent of survivors had clinical sequelae, half of which prevented normal adaptation to social life. With Hib meningitis, 27 per cent of children died and 38 per cent of survivors had clinical sequelae, a quarter of which prevented normal adaptation to social life[19]. Hib meningitis and (the less prevalent) meningococcal meningitis are vaccine preventable. There is currently no vaccine for pneumococcal meningitis.

Neurological problems can also be caused by other forms of encephalitis. This is an inflammation of the brain caused primarily by viral infections and can lead to seizures, cognitive and motor disabilities, coma and blindness in survivors. A vaccine exists for Japanese encephalitis virus which is the leading cause of encephalitis in Asia. Clearly, many infections in early childhood have a severe impact on children's mental and physical abilities and have long-term effects on their chances of attending school.

The impact of school-age health and nutrition on enrolment

Diseases in infancy and early childhood, considered in the previous section, affect school enrolment largely through the severe effects they have on physical or mental development of children. Less severe conditions of poor health and nutrition can affect access to education at the time of enrolment.

Enrolment is delayed for children of short stature

A number of studies across Asia and Africa have found that stunted children (those with a low height-for-age) enrol in school later than other children[20-23]. This relationship is illustrated in Figure 3.1. Children are grouped according to the number of years they are lagging behind their peers at school. Those who have the appropriate age for their grade have an age-for-grade score of zero. Those who are a year older than the appropriate age for their grade have an age-for-grade z-score of -1, and so on. Children with a negative age-for-grade score were most likely those who enrolled late in school. The figure shows that more children are stunted (low height-for-age) among children who are too old for their grade.

Children who are behind in their schooling in both Ghana and Tanzania, are more likely to be stunted[23]. This relationship may be because poorer children are both more likely to be stunted and also more likely to be enrolled in school later. However, evidence from an external cause of nutritional deficit (a sudden change in cost of living in Pakistan, leading to a poorer diet) suggests that late enrolment is actually a consequence of stunting and not just a co-occurring consequence of poverty[24]. Furthermore, whereas poor children are often found to forgo schooling to engage in economic activities such as fishing or farming, a study in Tanzania[25] found that stunted children were less likely to engage in these activities as well as being less likely to enrol in school.

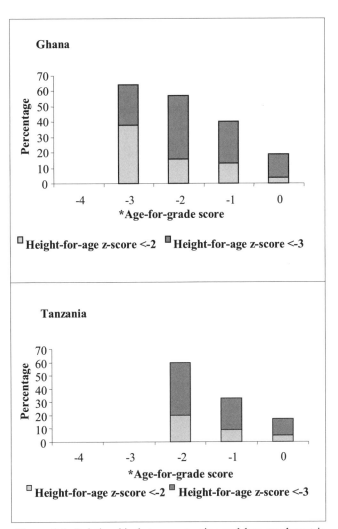

Figure 3.1. Relationship between stunting and late enrolment in schoolchildren from Ghana and Tanzania. *Age-for-grade score = number of years behind in schooling. *Source* Partnership for Child Development (1999)[23].

Child health affects parental enrolment decisions

It is likely that the delayed enrolment of undernourished children, discussed above, results from parental perceptions of their children's suitability for schooling and other activities. Smaller children are perceived as physically and perhaps mentally immature: anecdotal reports from several African countries suggest that children are considered ready for school when they are able to reach over their heads and touch one ear with the opposite arm, something determined by their physical stature. It may also reflect concerns about smaller children being able to walk safely over the long distances that are typical of journeys to school in the rural areas of many poor countries. Another factor that may explain the relationship between stunting and school enrolment is that parents consider investing in healthy children's education as most cost-effective and thus these children are prioritised above their less healthy siblings when decisions about school enrolment are made. Both of these explanations are consistent with the finding that the school enrolment of girls is delayed more by stunting than for boys[24], presumably reflecting parents' fragile resolve to invest in girls' education or their unwillingness in allowing young girls to walk long distances to school. Whatever the explanation, the finding that girls are differentially disadvantaged is of concern, given international targets to eliminate gender disparities in access to education in the next few years.

While taller children benefit from early enrolment, their stature may work against them later on in their education. Evidence from Peru[26] suggests that taller children drop-out of school earlier, possibly because they are perceived by their parents as adults who should no longer be in school.

The notion that parents are reluctant to invest in educating the least healthy of their children could apply equally to other conditions affecting children of school-age. There is limited information about other problems of health and nutrition affecting school enrolment. One study in Zanzibar found that out-of-school children were twice as likely to be infected with helminths than their in-school peers[27]. Another study in Tanzania found that out-of-school children were more wasted (a low weight for their height) and more anaemic than children in school[28]. However, in both of these cases it is not clear whether the health of children influenced their school enrolment or that both were consequences of poverty.

Overall, school enrolment suffers a great deal from the effects of health and nutrition. These range from severe effects on physical and mental development to more subtle effects involving the influence of child health on parental enrolment decisions. Once children do enrol in school, poor health and nutrition continues to affect their education by increasing absenteeism. This is considered in the next section.

Summary: Health, nutrition and school enrolment

- Poor health and nutrition in infancy and early childhood can lead to physical and mental disabilities which affect school enrolment, particularly where schools do not have facilities to cater for special needs.
- The most common nutritional cause of mental disabilities is iodine deficiency, which can cause severe mental retardation. Folate deficiency in pregnancy leads to spina bifida, causing motor disability in around 0.1 per cent of live births. Every year, vitamin A deficiency causes 350,000 new cases of blindness or partial blindness in children.
- Early childhood stunting has long-term effects on children's enrolment, absenteeism and grade repetition at primary school.
- Malaria is the most common infectious disease causing mental disability in low income countries. Protection from malaria in early childhood may lead to increased enrolment for girls.
- Mental disability also results from rubella and syphilis infections during pregnancy and from meningitis and encephalitis in young children. Polio infection leads to physical disabilities but has been eradicated from almost all countries.
- Stunted school-age children enrol later in school than their peers.

Absenteeism and drop-out

Absenteeism is perhaps the first educational effect of poor health and nutrition that comes to mind. In poor countries, repeated absenteeism is a particular concern because it can eventually lead to drop-out from school. Many forms of ill health lead to children being absent from school. We consider first the infectious diseases leading to absenteeism and then the diseases of poor nutrition.

Malaria prevention improves school attendance

Malaria has been identified as a major cause of school absenteeism. Around 40 per cent of the world's population is at risk of malaria infection, so any impact the disease has on education is likely to be far-reaching. In Kenya, it was found that primary school students miss 11 per cent of school days per year because of malaria, and secondary school students miss 4.3 per cent of school days[29]. A study in Senegal found that malaria accounted for 36 per cent of school absences due to medical reasons during the high transmission season[30].

Such studies are likely to understate the impact of malaria on education because they have not considered the cumulative impact of repeated absenteeism over several years. School-age children suffer around 0.25 and 2.3 malaria attacks a year[31] and thus the cumulative effect of these attacks on school attendance may be sufficient to cause children to repeat grades at school and eventually to drop out entirely. In addition, malaria attacks in children of preschool age, who bear the greatest burden of the malaria disease, may lead to increased absenteeism among their elder school-age sisters, who are often called upon to stay at home and look after younger siblings.

Oral antimalarial treatment can be administered to prevent the disease. Work in Ghana in the 1950s was successful in reducing school absenteeism by 50 per cent using this method[32]. A recent study in Sri Lanka[33] found a 3.4 per cent reduction in absenteeism – a 62.5 per cent reduction in absenteeism due to malaria – after regular treatment with chloroquine. However, concerns over cost and emerging resistance of the parasite to drugs has led to a preference for prompt diagnosis and treatment – rather than prevention through drug treatment – as a means of reducing the morbidity related to the disease[31]. Encouraging children to sleep under insecticide-treated bednets can also be effective in reducing the incidence of malaria[34].

Deworming improves school attendance

Worm infections are also known to increase absenteeism from school. Roundworm infections in Jamaica were found to be related to school absenteeism in one study[35] and, in another study, the number of days missed from school was found to increase in proportion to the intensity of infection with another worm – whipworm[36] (see figure 3.2). A similar relationship was found for schistosomiasis (bilharzia) infection in Mali[37].

Treatment for worms is cheap and effective and involves a single oral dose of either albendazole or mebendazole for intestinal worms and praziquantel for bilharzias. Treatment can be effective in improving school attendance. In Jamaica, treatment against roundworm was found to improve the school attendance of children who had been infected with this worm and who were also stunted (a low height for their age, indicating poor nutritional status)[38]. Attendance was initially around 60 per cent and improved by 6.7 per cent after the deworming programme. In Kenya, schoolchildren who were given treatment against worms (hookworm and bilharzias) recorded improvements in school participation (a combined measure of enrolment and attendance)[39]. In the first year of treatment, participation was increased by 7 per cent (from a baseline of around 75 per cent participation). In the second year of treatment the increase in participation was slightly smaller at 4 per cent. The conclusion from these studies is that deworming is an effective way to improve school attendance.

School attendance is likely to be affected by many other infections but little evidence of this is documented. Other likely causes of absenteeism include acute respiratory infections, such as a simple cold or cough, otitis media, sore throat, laryngitis, bronchitis, or pneumonia, and diarrhoeal diseases. We now turn to nutritional diseases and their impact on attendance of both preschools and primary schools.

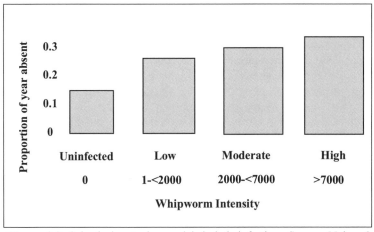

Figure 3.2. School absenteeism and helminth infection. *Source:* Nokes & Bundy (1993)[36].

Improved nutrition increases attendance at preschools

Two recent studies provide examples of how programmes to improve children's nutritional status can have beneficial effects on attendance of preschool institutions. One study in informal settlements in East Delhi gave a course of iron supplementation and deworming treatment to children attending preschools run by women from the local community. Attendance of the preschools rose by 5.8 per cent from levels of around 70 per cent representing a one-fifth reduction in absenteeism[40]. A school feeding programme in Kenya also found improvements in attendance as a result of the intervention. The programme offered children a cup of porridge for breakfast. School participation was 35.9 per cent where meals were provided and 27.4 per cent in comparison schools, indicating an improvement in attendance of around one-third. Improvements in participation resulted both from attracting new children to the school and by improving the attendance of children already enrolled. It is likely that attendance improved due to the incentive to attend provided by the school breakfast, rather than as a result of improved health of children[41].

School feeding programmes improve primary school attendance

Earlier in this chapter we saw how stunting affected children's chances of being enrolled. Nutritional status is also related to children's attendance once they are enrolled in school[42]. However, it is difficult to establish the reason for this and a likely explanation is that stunted children come from poorer households whose children have poorer school attendance in any case.

School feeding programmes are often proposed as a way of encouraging children to attend school. However, few evaluations have determined whether or not this is the case. One study in Jamaica[43] gave breakfast to children for a year and found that attendance rose by 2.3 per cent from a baseline of around 80 per cent. It is not clear whether this improvement is achieved because the feeding programmes improve children's health or because the food acts as an incentive for them to attend school. It is important to make this distinction when comparing school feeding programmes with other policies to increase access, such as other health interventions and conditional cash transfers. If school feeding is merely an incentive to attend school, cash incentives may be a more efficient way of achieving the same end.

The relationship between micronutrient deficiencies and school attendance has not been investigated extensively. However, one study in Jamaica found that anaemic children were less likely to attend school than non-anaemic children[35].

At least one study has been successful in improving school attendance via a combination of feeding and micronutrient supplementation. In South Africa, absenteeism related to diarrhoea and respiratory infections among primary schoolchildren was reduced as a result of a year of receiving biscuits fortified with iron, iodine and beta-carotene (a precursor to vitamin A)[44]. The improvement in attendance was substantial. Diarrhoea-related absenteeism fell from 79 days to 52 days. If we assume a school year of around 180 days, this represents a fall in absenteeism from 44 per cent to 29 per cent – an increase in attendance of 15 per cent. This is a larger increase than for other interventions discussed in this section and supports our argument that improving health and nutrition can have a substantial impact on education.

In conclusion, there are several programmatic options for increasing children's attendance through improved health and nutrition. Deworming, malaria prevention and school feeding have the clearest impacts on attendance.

Parental infection with HIV&AIDS leads to absenteeism

The previous sections of this chapter looked at how a child's health and nutrition can affect their chances of school enrolment and their school attendance thereafter. In addition, the health and nutrition of those around them can affect their schooling. Girls may be required to stay at home to care for siblings who are unwell. When parents become ill, children may be required to carry out parental duties that prevent them from going to school. Prolonged ill health in the family can affect the household income which has knock-on effects for children's chances of going to school.

The impact of family and community health on children's schooling will be more acute when more members of the community are afflicted. Seasonal diseases such as malaria, other epidemics and famines are thus particularly likely to disrupt children's schooling.

There is increasing evidence of the impact the HIV&AIDS pandemic is having on children's schooling. Children from AIDS-afflicted families suffer from the stigma attached to the disease, with some children turned away from school. However, the disease probably has its greatest effect on children's education when one or more parents die. In Kenya, children's school attendance dropped by 9 per cent in the year after a maternal death and 4 per cent after a paternal death[45]. In Malawi, 9.1 per cent of children were found to drop-out of school the year following the death of one parent. Those who had lost both parents were twice as likely to drop-out, with 17.1 per cent of children leaving school in the following year[46]. In Tanzania, the primary school enrolment of maternal orphans was delayed, although they were not more likely to drop-out of school once enrolled[47]. In Zimbabwe, orphanhood was found to decrease the likelihood of school completion, due to gaps in support from the extended family. However, school completion was sustained – particularly for female orphans – where orphanhood resulted in a female-headed household and greater access to external resources[48].

Summary: Health, nutrition and school attendance

- Both iron supplementation and school feeding programmes have been shown to improve attendance at preschools.
- The clearest evidence for improvements in primary school attendance comes from malaria prevention programmes, deworming programmes and school feeding programmes.
- Loss of one or both parents due to HIV&AIDS can lead to delayed enrolment, reduced attendance and increased drop-out.

Interventions: What works?

In considering which interventions are effective in improving access to school we will focus on those that can be delivered through school-based programmes. This is because school health and nutrition programmes are the focus of this book and because the best evidence is available for these types of interventions.

Table 3.1 summarises the effectiveness of the interventions for which evidence is available. School feeding, malaria prevention and deworming have all been effective in improving school attendance with increases ranging from 2 to 7 per cent. One study found a decrease in diarrhoea-related absenteeism of 15 per cent due to a programme giving children fortified biscuits. This study did not report overall attendance so the figure may not be comparable.

Overall, improved health and nutrition appears to be an effective way of improving school participation. Increases of 2 to 7 per cent in attendance represent an additional 1 or 2 weeks spent at school per year.

Table 3.1. The effectiveness of evidence-based interventions on improving school attendance.

Study	Country	Intervention	Age (years)	Sample characteristics	Increase in attendance (%)
Feeding Powell et al. 1998[43]	Jamaica	Daily breakfast for 1 year	M=9		2.3
van Stuivenberg 2001[44]	South Africa	Fortified biscuits	6-11		15.0
Deworming Simeon et al. 1995[38]	Jamaica	Deworming	7-10	Mild-moderate whipworm	6.7*
Miguel & Kremer 2004[39]	Kenya	Deworming	6-18		7.0
Malaria Prevention Fernando et al. 2005[33]	Sri Lanka	Antimalaria pills (chloroquine)	6-12		3.4

*For children with poor nutritional status only.

Conclusion

In this chapter we have presented evidence of the ways in which poor health and nutrition can substantially affect children's education – by delaying enrolment, increasing absenteeism and precipitating drop-out. The range of studies surveyed illustrates two of the reasons for supporting health and nutrition programmes.

Disease affects education throughout childhood

We have seen how poor health and nutrition can affect access to schooling in infancy, early childhood, and in the school-age years. There is no specific window in which access to schooling is threatened by poor health and nutrition.

There is a potential for health and nutrition programmes to have a positive impact on access to education throughout childhood. Further weight is given to this argument when we consider the impact of health and nutrition on cognitive abilities and educational achievement in the next two chapters.

Improving children's health and nutrition brings substantial benefits for education

It is surprising how influential simple interventions – such as giving a deworming pill to children – can be on their education. In the studies we reported, health and nutrition interventions result in an additional 1 or 2 weeks spent at school per year. These studies possibly underestimate the overall effect on education. Much of the evidence discussed relates to one or two conditions in isolation, but it is likely that the poorest children suffer from a number of conditions, each exacerbating the effects of the other. Also, few studies have been able to track the long-term effects of illness on educational outcomes. As such, they fail to capture the chain of consequences that can be set off by ill health at one point in a child's education, the vicious circle of underachievement that can be triggered by ill health and other adverse events. For example, absenteeism leads to poor performance which increases the chances of children being required to repeat a year of schooling. This increases the financial cost of education for the children's parents and erodes faith in the education system. Both of these factors in turn increase the likelihood of the child dropping out of school. Children's attendance in the first year of school in particular may have a long-lasting effect. One study in South Africa found that children's educational achievement in the first year of schooling was a crucial predictor of the likelihood of having to repeat grades later on (and thus, presumably, the likelihood of dropping out of school)[49]. This study also highlights the ways in which cognitive function and school attendance can interact (and we discuss further its implications in Chapter 6). Children with poor cognitive abilities are less likely to be able to cope with the adverse effects of missing school through illness. This interaction is particularly important to consider within the context of this book as the same illnesses that affect school enrolment can also impair children's cognitive functions. These effects on cognitive function, and also on educational achievement, are considered in the next two chapters.

Chapter 4

Long-term effects of preschool health and nutrition on educational achievement

In this chapter and in Chapter 5 we consider the effects of health and nutrition on behaviour and cognitive function – especially those that are essential for schooling. In doing so, we further illustrate the two arguments for health and nutrition programmes that were introduced in Chapter 3. Many examples in the current chapter support the first of these arguments that disease affects education throughout childhood. The current chapter shows how education benefits from good nutrition in pregnancy, infancy and early childhood. Furthermore, we argue against the idea of a critical period for the educational benefits of good nutrition. There is no sense in which health and nutrition programmes miss the boat if they are not implemented early in life. Interventions are effective through childhood. The current chapter also provides examples to support our argument that improved health and nutrition has a large impact on educational outcomes. Treating iron deficient infants improves their mental development by the equivalent of around 20 IQ points; malaria prevention in early childhood results in children staying at primary school for a year longer. These are both substantial improvements from a simple health or nutrition intervention.

Two further arguments to support health and nutrition programmes are introduced in this chapter. In support of the first of these arguments, we will see how improved health and nutrition brings the greatest benefits to the poor and disadvantaged: education of the poor benefits more from nutritional supplements, girls' enrolment benefits most from malaria prevention and the cognitive development of low birth weight babies benefits most from breast-feeding. The second argument for health and nutrition programmes introduced in this chapter is that health and education reinforce one another. We will see how programmes to stimulate young children's cognitive development work hand-in-hand with

48 ©CAB International 2008. *School Health, Nutrition and Education for All: Levelling the Playing Field (*M.C.H. Jukes *et al.)*

nutritional supplementation, and how cognitive delays of undernourished children can be reversed only by a combination of early childhood education and nutritional supplements.

In this chapter we look at how these arguments apply first to nutritional deficiencies in young children and then to infectious diseases of early childhood. First, we look at the mechanisms by which poor health and nutrition affect the mental development of children.

Mechanisms for the effects of health and nutrition on learning

The ways in which health and nutrition can affect behaviour are complex and it will be helpful to consider these before analysing evidence for the effects of specific diseases on behaviour. The next two sections look at the mechanisms by which diseases can directly and indirectly affect behavioural development.

Direct effects of health and nutrition on behaviour

The most apparent effects are those that directly affect the central nervous system. Mechanisms for these effects are discussed in more detail later on in the chapter and are summarised here. Nutritional deficiencies affect the brain in several ways[1] corresponding to the many elements of a brain's complex system (see Box 4.1). Neurotransmitter function can be affected by changes in nutritional intake leading in some cases to long-term impairment of neurotransmitter systems. Similarly, the electrical signals generated by neurons can also be affected by nutritional deficiencies. Changes in brain structure can also ensue from nutritional deficiencies, particularly those occurring during important periods of brain growth. Although many nutritionally induced structural changes recover after nutritional health is restored, some alterations are permanent.

The introduction of foreign bodies or toxic substances to the central nervous system can be as damaging as a reduction in the supply of essential nutrients. For example, the cerebral malaria parasite, *Plasmodium falciparum,* and the eggs of the schistosome parasite (also known as bilharzia) can both disrupt the supply of oxygen and nutrients to the brain[2,3]. Other parasites living outside the central nervous system release substances to facilitate their feeding or to suppress immune response or digestion by the host. These secretions may enter the central nervous system and affect brain function[3].

Indirect effects of health and nutrition on behaviour

In addition to the primary effects of illness, secondary behavioural consequences may emerge with time. Here we mean that direct effects on one type of behaviour influence the development of another type of behaviour. This is particularly true in early childhood when there is a high interdependency between physical, emotional and mental development. For example, iron deficient children are often more fearful and more likely to cling to their mothers[4]. Consequently these children do not explore and interact with their environment to the same extent. This kind of interactive exploration of the environment is essential for children's mental development. It is how children learn. So, a secondary consequence of being more fearful is that children fail to learn about the world they live in – the people and things they interact with – and their social and cognitive development is delayed. Similarly, damage to (bodily) muscles may affect the long-term (mental) ability to control movement; impairment of sensory organs can affect perceptual and other higher-order cognitive functions.

Box 4.1. Basic processes of the brain

Poor health and nutrition affect the basic processes of the brain, how electrical signals are passed on from one cell to another. The following is a brief summary of this communication process highlighting terms that crop up in the main text.

The brain is made up of a dense network of cells, most of which constitutes supporting tissue known as *glial cells*. Around 10 per cent of cells are *neurons* – cells designed to carry electrical signals. Electrical signals pass along *axons* which branch out to reach other neurons. In between the axons of connecting neurons is a gap, called a *synapse*. Electrical signals result in chemicals, known as *neurotransmitters*, being released into the synapse. Neurotransmitters bind onto *receptors* in the adjacent neuron initiating another electrical signal. And so electrical activity spreads. As the brain develops, axons become sheathed in a fatty insulation called *myelin*. Myelin increases the speed of electrical conduction. Myelinisation of the brain takes several years and is not complete in some regions of the brain until after puberty.

Source: Kandel, Schwartz and Jessell (2001)[5].

Indirect effects can also extend to caregivers. For example, parents have been observed to interact less frequently with children who are severely malnourished[6]. This lack of stimulation may in turn affect children's development.

Indirect effects may be common in older children too. For example, the primary effects of parasitic worm infections may be to cause discomfort and affect a child's concentration in class. The secondary consequences of this will be that the child learns less in class. A treatment for the infection may remove discomfort and improve concentration but cannot compensate for lost learning.

This discussion highlights the importance of understanding the effect of disease on cognitive abilities. The mechanisms for these effects have implications for how they should be treated. In some cases the effects of a disease may be irreversible, for example, when the supply of nutrients is reduced during critical periods of brain growth. In such cases, prevention is better than cure. In other cases, the primary effects of a disease, such as mental fatigue, may be immediately reversible while secondary symptoms remain. There are also instances where secondary symptoms can be treated separately. For example, children infected with worms who have fallen behind in class because they are unable to concentrate, will benefit from deworming treatment to remove parasites and improve concentration (the primary effect), but may also require remedial teaching to compensate for months or years of impaired learning (the secondary effects). In fact, some problems can be addressed effectively by tackling the secondary consequences directly, bypassing the primary effects of a disease. Later in this chapter we will see that teaching a mother to stimulate the mind of an undernourished child can have a greater long-term effect on their development than giving them supplements to improve their nutritional status.

In the following sections we will look at specific conditions, first of poor nutrition, and second of infectious disease. These sections will consider direct effects on the brain, effects on behaviour in the short term, and how these effects have long-term consequences for children's performance in school.

Nutritional deficiencies and child development

Children can suffer many different nutritional deficits before reaching school-age. Undernutrition and iron deficiency anaemia are the most common conditions and many studies have examined the impact of these conditions on brain and behaviour. These studies form the bulk of the following sections before we consider less studied conditions in this age group – deficiencies of iodine and zinc.

Undernutrition

Undernutrition (also called 'protein energy malnutrition') is a general term applied to children with heights and weights below age-referenced criteria resulting from insufficient protein or calories in their diet. This is contrasted with our use of the term 'malnutrition' which refers to diets that have sufficient calories but lack essential elements, such as micronutrients. Undernutrition typically results from a severe or chronic lack of a range of essential nutrients rather than from just a lack of protein. This complicates the discussion of the cognitive consequences of undernutrition because several different causal factors may be involved, each potentially associated with a different means of affecting brain and behaviour.

Box 4.2. Brain and behaviour

"Men ought to know that from the brain, and from the brain only, arise our pleasures, joys, laughter and jests, as well as our sorrows, pains, griefs and tears."

Hippocrates[7]

The brain is often described in lay terms as having a role in cognitive processing but not in other less intellectual behaviours. The brain is for thinking but not for feeling. Emotions exists somewhere in the body outside the brain. This is evident in the language we use to describe our behaviours. Complex reasoning is described as a 'cerebral' activity undertaken by 'brainy' people whereas instincts and emotions are 'gut' reactions. Tension between rational and emotional approaches to problems are characterised as being between the head and the heart.

In fact, this conception has more to do with where these phenomena are experienced (thinking makes the head hurt, joy makes the heart leap) than where they originate. All movements, emotions, intuitions, thoughts and instincts, in short all behaviours, are controlled by the brain. It is important to understand this when approaching the discussions in the present chapter and in Chapter 5. For example, we present evidence that iron deficiency has a direct effect on the brain. This does not imply that iron deficiency necessarily affects the cognitive processes of reasoning, perception and memory – the 'cerebral activities'. Because the brain controls all behaviours, impairment to the physical brain can lead to disruption of any of the set of human behaviours and emotions.

Levels of description

It is also important to recognise that brain activity and behaviours are alternative descriptions of the same phenomenon. Every observable behaviour or thought process takes place at the same time as an associated activity in the brain. Thus, brain and behaviour represent two levels of describing the same phenomenon but not two different phenomena. Understanding this will help in interpreting the literature reviewed in the following two chapters. Some studies focus on changes in the brain. Implicit in the discussion of such studies is that there is a related change in behaviour, whether or not this has been identified. Similarly, studies that focus on changes in behaviour recognise that an associated change will have taken place in the brain. Thus, descriptions in terms of brain and behaviour should be seen as complementary and not in competition.

Undernutrition affects many aspects of brain development

Brain growth is resistant to the effects of undernutrition relative to the rest of the body. Initially, the brain is spared the growth retardation resulting from lack of nutrients. But when nutritional deficiencies become sufficiently severe, growth processes in all areas of the brain are affected[8]. This includes those growth processes that are taking place at the time of the nutritional deficiency and some that take place afterwards, as a result of a cascade of effects[9]. It has often been hypothesised that nutritional deficiencies are more likely to have permanent effects on the brain if they occur during critical periods of brain growth. However, brain structure typically recovers after nutritional disease is treated (e.g. by nutritional supplementation). Some brain areas do not recover from nutritional insults in some circumstances: these include the hippocampus (involved in memory and learning) and the cerebellum (associated with balance, movement and posture).

The specific impacts of nutritional deficiencies on brain development are many[1]. Short and long-term changes in diet can affect the function of neurotransmitters (chemicals that transmit signals between neurons). More severe nutritional deficiencies can have lasting effects on behaviour due to effects on synthesis of neurotransmitters, the process by which transmitters are broken down (neurotransmitter degradation) and on the receptor sites where neurotransmitters bind to neurons. Low protein diets in young rats later affect the electrophysiological response of the hippocampus, correlated with behavioural changes. Changes in neuroanatomy resulting from nutritional deficiencies include retarded acquisition of myelin (fatty insulation for neuronal axons, increasing speed of signal transmission) and glial cells (cells that support the tissue of the central nervous system).

Much of the above research on nutrition and the brain has been conducted on rats. The behavioural correlates of impaired brain development in humans are poorly understood. However, overall behavioural effects of nutritional deficiencies in childhood have been reasonably well characterised and are summarised in the following sections. (See Box 4.2 for a description of how brain and behaviour are related.)

Behavioural development is delayed in undernourished children

Evidence suggests that undernutrition is associated with poor mental development in the early years. A low height-for-age or low weight-for-age is associated with impairment in developmental levels of young children[10]. For example, in Guatemala the length and weight of 1 and 2 year olds was related to their scores on a test on infant mental development[11]. In Kenya, undernourished infants were found to be less sociable than adequately nourished infants[12].

In addition to the effect of chronic malnutrition, acute episodes of severe malnutrition (typically <60 per cent reference weight-for-age) bring about characteristic changes in behaviour[13]. Affected children show increased apathy, decreased activity and explore their environment less frequently and less thoroughly. After the acute episode, all behaviours return to normal, except for the children's thoroughness of exploration of their environment. Developmental levels are lower in hospitalised children with severe malnutrition, but not more so than in children hospitalised for other reasons[14].

Similarly, on recovery the development levels of severely malnourished children remain impaired, but this is likely attributable to chronic undernutrition rather than the acute episode itself[15].

Box 4.3. Demonstrating that poor cognitive function is *caused* by poor health and nutrition

The impact of disease on cognitive function can often be difficult to infer from data. Healthy individuals are less likely to be poor than those suffering ill health or poor nutrition of one form or another. The poorest members of society have fewer opportunities to develop their minds. This is true both at school, where teaching is likely to be of low quality, and at home, where they have fewer toys and books and where their parents have lower levels of education, and have lower expectations for their children's education. The poor are also likely to suffer from other diseases and to have suffered from poor health in the past. In short, there are many ways in which poverty can lead to poor cognitive abilities.

Studies that merely observe children's health and their cognitive function are unable to demonstrate that one causes the other. A study may show that children who are undernourished also tend to have poorer cognitive function, but it doesn't follow that undernutrition causes poor cognitive function. Both may result from a third factor, such as poverty. Here, poverty is termed as a 'confounding' factor. It is possible to control statistically for confounding factors such as poverty and other illnesses, but causality can only be demonstrated by treating a randomly selected group of children for a disease (and not treating others) and observing changes in cognitive function. Such experiments are called randomised controlled trials. In this way, changes in cognitive function can be reliably attributed to the treatment of the disease. However, it is possible that treating a disease will not reverse the cognitive deficits it causes. Thus, a failure to find a treatment effect in such studies cannot be reliably interpreted as evidence that there are no cognitive consequences of the disease.

The most effective way to demonstrate the effect of a disease on cognition and education is to conduct a prospective randomised controlled trial. Here, a group of participants is given some measures to prevent disease, and these are then compared to a second group which received no such prevention measures. In such cases, differences in cognitive function between the two groups can be reliably attributed to the disease. However, such studies are relatively rare in the field because measures with proven health benefits cannot be ethically withheld from children. Thus, many studies cannot be conducted with adequate control groups and results are often difficult to interpret.

Preventing nutritional deficiency promotes cognitive development

Quality evidence of the relationship between nutrition and cognitive development comes from intervention trials (see Box 4.3) that fall into two categories: preventive and therapeutic. We will look at these in turn. With infants and preschool children, preventive supplementary feeding can have a significant impact on development. In many countries, steps have been taken to prevent malnutrition in children by beginning nutritional supplementation in pregnancy and continuing in infancy. This approach has been successful in improving the motor development of infants in Taiwan by 8 months of age[16]. In Guatemala, a similar supplementation programme found small improvements in cognitive function for children between 3 and 7 years[17].

Supplementation in Mexico from shortly after birth and throughout the first 3 years was found to improve children's school performance, language, motor skills, adaptive behaviour and personal and social behaviour[18]. In addition, from 8 months of age, supplemented children became increasingly active and by 2 years of age were showing eight times more activity than non-supplemented children. A similar programme with high-risk mothers in Bogotá, Colombia was successful in improving the mental and – to a greater extent – motor development of their children at 18 months and also their language skills at 36 months[19]. One group of mothers in this study received education on how to stimulate cognitive development in their children. This programme improved children's personal/social skills and language at 18 months and language only at 36 months. In addition, the nutritional supplementation and maternal education programme worked synergistically. In other words, supplementation improved the effectiveness of stimulation, or vice versa, such that the benefit of receiving both interventions was greater than the sum of the independent benefits of the two interventions. This illustrates one of our arguments for health and nutrition programmes introduced in Chapter 1: health and education reinforce one another. A final finding is worthy of note from this study: overall, girls benefited more from the programme than boys. This effect is consistent with another thesis of this book – that health interventions have the greatest impact for the most disadvantaged groups in society. This particular finding suggests that improved health and nutrition may be an effective way towards reaching the gender equity goals of Education for All.

One study in Kenya[20] found a benefit of a school feeding programme for children's educational outcomes. Children were given a breakfast meal through an ECD class and improvement was found in educational achievement, but not in tests of cognitive function, and was only evident in classes with an experienced teacher. The improvement in educational achievement was around 0.4 SD (see Box 4.4 for an explanation of effect sizes expressed in SD units).

The four preventive studies reported above were all of significant duration (>2 years). A short-term study in West Java[21] demonstrated that it is possible to find improvements in the motor development of children after only 90 days of supplementation, beginning after pregnancy at between 6 and 20 months of age.

Nutritional supplements and psychosocial stimulation help reverse cognitive delays

Results from therapeutic trials also provide strong evidence of a link between nutritional supplementation and cognitive development. These studies have typically involved remedial nutritional supplementation of malnourished children. In Bogotá, Colombian children from a poor urban area who underwent four periods of an educational stimulation and nutritional supplementation programme, between the ages of 42 and 84 months, showed a gain in general cognitive ability of 0.80 SD in comparison with a group who received the same treatment for only one period between the ages of 74 and 84 months[22]. In so doing, these children closed the gap in IQ between themselves and a group of richer urban children. In this programme, all beneficiaries received both nutritional supplements and education so it is not possible to decipher which of these two interventions was most influential in improving children's cognitive abilities. A more recent study in Jamaica helped resolve this issue by giving poor, urban and undernourished children aged between 9 and 24 months a 2 year programme of either nutritional supplements, stimulations, both interventions, or neither intervention. The gains in overall development quotient (DQ; an IQ equivalent for infants and young children), were impressive and further supports our argument that, improving children's health and nutrition brings substantial benefits for children's development. Nutritional supplementation accounted for an increase of 6.1 DQ points (0.66 SD) over 2 years, while stimulation improved DQ by 7.3 points (0.79 SD). Larger gains were found for the motor development – 12.4 DQ points (1.04 SD) due to supplementation and 10.3 DQ points (0.87 SD) due to stimulation. Similar effects were seen with other dimensions of child development. The effects of the two interventions were additive (receiving both interventions was better than receiving only one of them) but there was no interaction between them (nutritional supplementation did not improve the effectiveness of the stimulation programme, for example). Significantly, the children who did receive both treatments effectively closed the gap in DQ between themselves and adequately nourished children[23]. Slightly larger effects were found in the Jamaica studies for a long-term programme of psychosocial stimulation to promote the development of severely malnourished young children[24]. After 6 months, children who had received the stimulation programme were around 15 DQ points (~1 SD) better off than the control group. Participants in both of these studies in Jamaica have been followed up for a number of years. Results from these studies constitute a substantial part of the evidence for a long-term impact of poor nutrition on cognitive development, considered in the next section.

Box 4.4. How big an impact?

Hundreds of studies are reported in this book. They were conducted in almost as many different settings and were assessed using a wide variety of cognitive and educational achievement measures. We need to draw comparisons among them. But how does a 10 point improvement on Jamaican versions of an intelligence test compare with a 5 point improvement in a language test in Indonesia?

The approach taken throughout this book is to report such improvements in units of standard deviations (SDs). This allows comparability across tests. The standard deviation is a measure of the variability in scores. Expressing improvements in units of standard deviations gives you an idea of how the change in test scores compares to the overall range in scores. This is illustrated in the figure with the case of IQ scores – a frequently reported outcome in this book. IQ scores are distributed in the same way as most test scores – in a bell-shaped curve, with many children scoring around the mid-point and many fewer with very low or very high scores. For such a distribution of scores (known as the normal distribution) it turns out that the highest scores are always around 3 standard deviations higher than the mean; and the lowest scores are around 3 standard deviations lower than the mean. So when studies report an improvement of 1 SD following a nutritional intervention, this can be thought of as raising scores from the mean to around a third of the way towards the highest scores. This is true whatever the type of test being considered.

In the case of the IQ test, the standard deviation is 15. As shown on the graph, almost everyone has an IQ below 145 (3 SD above the mean). An intervention that improves intelligence test scores by 1 SD is equivalent to a 15 point improvement in IQ – or raising someone at mean level a third of the way towards the highest IQs (145).

Effect sizes are reported in units of standard deviation throughout the book – because a 1 SD improvement means the same for any test score. We have used SD units wherever original studies reported these statistics or else presented sufficient data to allow calculation of these statistics.

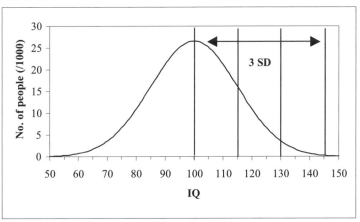

Undernutrition affects cognitive abilities in the long term

It is clear that undernutrition affects the mental development of young children and that both nutritional supplements and psychosocial stimulation can improve the development of undernourished children. What implications does this have for the child's schooling and their ability to learn in the school-age years? A study in Kenya[12] found some continuity in the cognitive development of undernourished children which would suggest that deficits in infancy are carried through at least to preschool age. Children who were undernourished at 6 months were also less sociable, and those who were less sociable at 6 months had lower development scores at 30 months and poorer verbal comprehension scores at 5 years.

The long-term effects of severe malnutrition

There is more direct evidence that undernutrition has a long-term impact on cognitive development. Beginning with the most profound nutritional insults, severe malnutrition in early childhood has a long-term effect on development. Children in Jamaica who had suffered from severe malnutrition between the ages of 6 and 24 months were found to lag behind adequately nourished children who had been hospitalised for other reasons at ages 7, 8, 9 and 14 on a range of IQ tests. At 14 years they were substantially delayed in overall IQ (1.50 SD below the control group), vocabulary (1.33 SD) and tests of educational achievement, even after accounting for differences in the background of the two groups of children[25]. These are substantial differences, which are not unique. More than a dozen other studies have found a relationship between severe malnutrition in early childhood and subsequent cognitive or behavioural problems up to adolescence[13].

There is potential for interventions to reduce the gap between severely undernourished children and their peers. The study in Jamaica found that a 3 year programme to teach mothers how to improve the development of their child (aged 6 to 24 months at the beginning of the programme) conferred significant long-term benefits to severely malnourished children. At age 14 the undernourished children whose mothers had taken part in the education programme were only 0.28 SD behind adequately nourished children on overall IQ scores and 0.68 SD ahead of undernourished children who had not taken part in the intervention[25].

The long-term effects of mild and moderate malnutrition

Severe malnutrition clearly has a substantial long-term effect on child development. Of potentially greater concern is the effect that mild and moderate malnutrition has on child development, given the high prevalence of this condition among children in poor countries. This issue has again been addressed by researchers in Jamaica who followed 127 undernourished children for 8 years. As discussed above, these children received a 2 year programme of nutritional supplementation psychosocial stimulation, both interventions, or neither intervention. Four years after the end of the interventions, perceptual/motor skills were superior in those children who had received stimulation[26]. The same skills were also superior for children who had originally received a nutritional supplement and whose mothers had the highest verbal intelligence. One explanation for this interaction was that the most intelligent mothers were also the ones giving children the most stimulation. There were no effects of the intervention on general cognitive abilities or on memory, although each intervention group had higher scores than the control subjects on more of these cognitive tests than would be expected by chance. Thus, stimulation, and to a lesser extent supplementation, had modest effects on children's cognitive abilities over 4 years.

The study also compared the stunted children taking part in the original intervention with other children from similar backgrounds, but who were known not to be stunted at the time of the interventions. These non-stunted children had higher scores on the general cognitive factor than previously stunted children, although were no better in perceptual/motor skills or memory.

There were similar findings 8 years after the end of the intervention. Children who received stimulation as infants had a higher IQ (by 0.42 SD) at ages 11 and 12 years while supplementation had no effect on cognitive abilities of children at this age. Again, children who were stunted before 2 years of age had a lower IQ (by 0.60 SD) and performed more poorly on 8 out of 9 cognitive tests (effect size range 0.38 SD to 0.61 SD) at age 11 and 12 years than children who were not stunted before 2 years of age[27]. These children were also more likely to have conduct disorders, and to perform poorly in arithmetic, spelling and reading tests[28]. Results of the Jamaica intervention studies are summarised in Figure 4.1.

The long-term effect of nutritional supplementation has also been investigated in other areas of the world. In Guatemala, children given nutritional supplements prenatally and in the immediate postnatal period (up to 2 years) were found to perform better as adolescents (aged 13 to 19 years) on tests of vocabulary, numeracy, knowledge and reading achievement[29]. Interestingly, these benefits were found only for those children of low socioeconomic status. This is another illustration of how health and nutrition programmes have the biggest impact for the poorest children. In tests of reading and vocabulary, the effect of supplements was most evident for children with the highest levels of education, further demonstrating that education and health work together. Performance in tests of memory and reaction time were also improved in supplemented children, although the improvement did not depend on socioeconomic status or education.

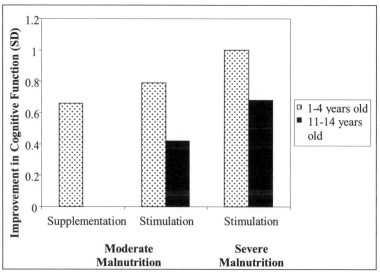

Figure 4.1. Summary of the Jamaica studies: immediate and long-term effects of nutritional supplementation and psychosocial stimulation on the cognitive development of children with moderate and severe malnutrition.

The studies in Jamaica and Guatemala show that a fairly sustained programme of nutritional supplementation and/or psychosocial stimulation, lasting for 2 years, can have long-term benefits for children's development. A study in Indonesia showed that even a 3 month programme of supplementation can have long-term effects[30]. Children supplemented before 18 months of age were found to have improved performance on a test of working memory at age 8, although no effect was observed on other measures of information processing, vocabulary, verbal fluency, arithmetic or tests of emotional response to a stressor. The conclusion from both of these studies is that fairly short periods of nutritional supplementation can have long-term effects on cognitive function.

Education and nutrition reinforce one another

The Jamaica studies showed how education interventions and nutrition interventions work together in improving children's development. A more recent study in Vietnam[31] adds to our understanding of the interaction between educational and nutritional interventions in early childhood. In this study, children aged from birth to 3 years in five communities, were given nutritional supplements. In two of these communities children took part in an ECD project at age 4 to 5 years. At age 6 to 8 years, those who had received both interventions scored 0.25 SD higher on the Raven's Progressive Matrices Test (a test of non-verbal reasoning) than those who had received only the nutritional intervention. The effect was particularly pronounced for those who were stunted at the time of testing. Among stunted children, those who had received both interventions scored significantly better (0.67 SD) than those who had only received the nutrition intervention. Furthermore, the ECD intervention appeared to cancel out the impact of stunting on cognitive abilities, whereas for those who had received nutritional supplements but no ECD intervention, there was a large (~0.5 SD) difference between stunted and non-stunted children (Figure 4.2).

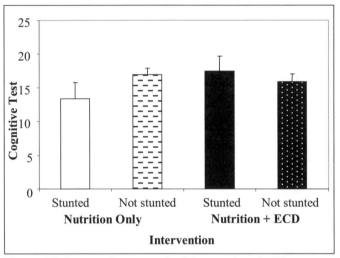

Figure 4.2. Impact of two preschool interventions in Vietnam on cognitive abilities of children aged 6 to 8 years. *Source:* Watanabe (2005)[31].

Nutrition affects cognitive development throughout childhood

We argued in Chapter 1 that health and nutrition programmes improve children's cognitive development and education throughout childhood. This is highlighted as an argument for health and nutrition programmes because it runs counter to received wisdom. The argument is particularly relevant to undernutrition. It might be expected that nutritional deficits in the first year of life have the greatest impact on development, or that in general, the earlier the intervention the better. However, evidence does not bear this out. A study in Colombia tried out different strategies for giving nutritional supplements to young children. In one group, supplements were given from the third trimester of pregnancy to 6 months after birth. A second group received supplements from 6 months to 3 years of age. The third group received supplements throughout – from pregnancy to 3 years of age. Results showed that supplementation in the latter period (6 months to 3 years) were most effective in improving cognitive development. There was no additional benefit for supplementation before and immediately after birth, and this early supplementation by itself was less effective than later supplementation[19]. A long-term study in the Philippines found that malnutrition in the second year of life actually had a stronger association with the performance of 8 year olds on a non-verbal test of intelligence than did malnutrition in the first year of life[32].

Other studies support early supplementation. The study from Indonesia, discussed above, found that children supplemented before, but not after 18 months of age, had improved performance on a test of working memory at age 8 years[30]. Another study in the Philippines found that children stunted in the first 6 months were more likely than those stunted later on, to have impaired cognitive performance at 8 years of age[33]. This however, was explained by the fact the children suffering the earliest bouts of malnutrition also suffered the most severe and persistent malnutrition. A confounding factor such as this is a reminder of the difficulty in interpreting findings related to timing effects of nutritional deficiencies on cognitive development (see Box 4.3). At present, there is no strong evidence that early (first year of life) interventions with children suffering from, or at risk of malnutrition, are more effective than interventions at a later age. It is likely that improved nutrition leads to improved development throughout childhood.

Mothers behave differently towards undernourished children

Not only is a child's behaviour affected by undernutrition, but a mother's behaviour is also related to the nutritional status of her child. In Egypt and in Kenya, maternal behaviour towards toddlers was found to be influenced more by the nutritional intake of the child than that of the mother[34]. Poorly nourished children are more likely to be carried by their mother and in general stay closer to their mother than adequately nourished children[6].

In addition to the effect child malnutrition has on maternal behaviour, evidence from Mexico suggests that mothers of malnourished children behave differently towards their children even before the onset of malnutrition[35]. They were less likely than other mothers to reward the successes of their child, were less affectionate and talked less to them. This could be because mothers of children who become malnourished are less well educated than other mothers[25]. In addition, mothers of malnourished children may often be poorly nourished themselves, which in turn affects their behaviour. In Kenya, it was found that although toddlers were protected from the effects of temporary food shortages, their mothers were not, and maternal nutritional deficiencies led to changes in the quality of mother-child interactions[36].

Whatever the explanation for the change in maternal behaviour, the implication is clear. We have seen that psychosocial stimulation is perhaps the most important factor in the prevention of poor cognitive outcomes in malnourished children. If these children typically receive poor levels of stimulation from their parents – for whatever reason – the lack of stimulation is likely to compound the effects of nutrition on their development.

Children with low birth weight have poor cognitive development

Undernutrition can affect cognitive development from before birth. Children with a low birth weight (LBW) or more generally, those born small for gestational age (SGA) have poor developmental outcomes in the long-term. Differences between SGA babies and those of normal birth weight typically do not appear in the first year of life[37], although this can depend on environmental factors. In Brazil, developmental delays were observed only in SGA babies who also received little stimulation in the home. Similarly, low birth weight affects infant development to a greater extent in the homes of illiterate mothers as compared to literate mothers. Deficits in developmental levels appear with high-risk infants in the second year with clear significant differences apparent by the third year. Some deficits were also found in the development levels of SGA babies between the ages of 4 and 7 years. A number of long-term studies have found cognitive deficits and poorer school performance in adolescents who were small for gestational age[38]. Only one such long-term study has been conducted in a poor country. This study found a small long-term effect of SGA on the mental performance of adolescent boys in India, but poor nutrition in early childhood had a greater impact on performance than SGA[39].

Children who are breast-fed have better cognitive abilities

The percentage of infants in least developed countries who are exclusively breast-fed in the first 6 months of life fell from 43 per cent in 1998 to 34 per cent in 2004[40]. In Western and Central Africa the figure is only 20 per cent. This is of concern, because breast-feeding is associated with a moderate long-term improvement in cognitive development. A review of 17 studies in rich countries estimated that breast-feeding led to an improvement of 3.2 IQ points (~0.21 SD), which was fairly stable across the lifespan from 3 to 50 years of age[41]. Low birth weight babies benefit most from breast-feeding, gaining 5.2 IQ points (0.35 SD) compared with a gain of 2.7 IQ points (0.18 SD) for children of normal birth weight. This reinforces our thesis, that the greatest benefits of good health and nutrition are seen in the most vulnerable children.

The length of breast-feeding is also important. Scandinavian children breast-fed for longer than 6 months were found to have improved cognitive test outcomes at 5 years compared with children who were breast-fed for less than 3 months[42]. However, it is difficult to be certain about such findings since mothers who choose to breast-feed are often more educated or more wealthy and this difference could explain some of the differences in IQ scores[43] although review studies do attempt to account for such factors in their estimates of IQ differences[41]. In general, the evidence is not conclusive, but is strongly suggestive of a link between breast-feeding and cognitive ability in later life.

Taken together, the evidence that undernutrition affects cognitive development is overwhelming. Poor nutrition in pregnancy, infancy and early childhood has immediate and long-term effects on cognitive abilities.

Summary: Undernutrition and child development

- The brain is initially spared the growth-retarding effects of undernutrition. Severe deficits do impair brain growth. In many, but not all cases, brain growth can recover.
- Undernourished children are less sociable and more apathetic than adequately nourished children. Mothers tend to carry poorly nourished children more often but give them less stimulation.
- Preventive nutritional supplementation beginning shortly after birth improves the cognitive development of young children.
- Developmental outcomes of severely malnourished children are poor. Encouraging psychosocial stimulation has a large impact (~1 SD) on developmental scores of these children. The benefits persist into adolescence.
- Moderate malnutrition also impairs cognitive development. Both psychosocial stimulation and nutritional supplementation can recover cognitive impairments in the short term, but only stimulation has a long-term effect.
- Stimulation and supplementation work together to improve cognitive development. Both may be needed for most effective rehabilitation.
- Nutritional supplementation in the first year of life is no more effective than later on in childhood in improving cognitive development.
- Breast-feeding and small for gestational age both have mild to moderate long-term effects on cognitive development.

Micronutrient deficiencies

Iron deficiency anaemia

We now consider a more specific case of poor nutrition – a deficiency in iron. In poor countries, children become deficient in iron because their diet is lacking in this micronutrient, because they fail to absorb iron from their diet or because infections, such as malaria or hookworm, cause loss of iron from the body. Iron is an important component of haemoglobin, the protein that fills red blood cells and transports oxygen around the body. Anaemia results when iron deficiency leads to a significant reduction in levels of haemoglobin. The following sections look at the impact of iron on the brain and then on behaviour.

Iron plays many different roles in the brain

Iron has many functions in the brain[44]. It is necessary for the production of myelin, the fatty coating around neurons that speeds the transmission of electrical signals; it facilitates the production of neurotransmitters, the chemicals that transmit messages between neurons; it is involved in the function of neuroreceptors, part of a neuron that receives the neurotransmitter's messages; and is essential for the metabolic processes that provide energy to the brain. The importance of iron for the brain varies between brain regions and also with age. For example, some regions of the human brain become iron rich only between 12 and 15 years of age.

Studies of rodents have improved our understanding of the effect of iron deficiency on the brain. A reduction in dietary iron of rodents quickly results in a reduction in brain iron. Levels of brain iron can be restored with supplementation but initial deficits may have irreversible effects on brain and behaviour. The damage caused by sustained periods of iron deficiency depends on the age of the individual and the stage of brain growth. For example, it is found that iron deficiency occurring during lactation depletes iron in a different region of the brain from iron deficiency later in life. Deficiency during the lactating period leads to permanent abnormalities in the production of one neurotransmitter and in behaviours associated with this neurotransmitter.

Similar studies cannot be conducted in humans. However, by recording electrical signals on the surface of skin, researchers have been able to show that neural conduction in the brain stem of iron deficient infants is slower than for iron replete infants[45]. Given the important role of iron in the brain, it is not surprising that iron deficiency leads to brain abnormalities. The next sections consider how these abnormalities manifest themselves as cognitive impairments.

Iron deficiency has a large impact on the mental development of children under 2 years

Evidence of the cognitive impact of iron deficiency is found to differ by age group[46]. It is a common finding that infants with iron deficiency have lower developmental levels than iron replete children. Lower scores on the Mental Development Index and the Psychomotor Development Index of the Bayley Scales of Infant Development have been found with 12 month old children in Chile[47], 12 to 23 month old children in Costa Rica[4], 6 to 24 month old children in Guatemala[48], and 12 to 18 month old children in Indonesia[49]. Iron deficiency anaemia also affects other aspects of infant behaviour. In the Costa Rica study[4], infants with iron deficiency anaemia were found to maintain closer contact with caregivers; to show less pleasure and delight; to be more wary, hesitant and easily tired; to make fewer attempts at test items; to be less attentive to instructions and demonstrations; and to be less playful. In addition, adults were found to behave differently towards iron deficient children, showing less affection and being less active in their interactions with these children. Such findings have serious implications for the amount of stimulation children receive, both from their own exploration of their environment and in the stimulation they receive from their caregivers. Such lack of stimulation is likely to affect children's long-term development, an issue to which we return in the following section.

What impact does iron supplementation have on the development of iron deficient children? Only one study has been conducted with children under 2 years of age in low income countries that has met rigorous criteria for experimental design (a double blind randomised controlled trial). This study in Indonesia[49] gave iron supplementation (iron sulphate) or a placebo to iron deficient children aged 12 to 18 months. Those receiving iron supplementation, showed impressive gains in the Bayley Scales of Infant Development. Their Mental Development Index rose by 19.3 DQ points (1.3 SD) and the Psychomotor Development score rose by 23.5 DQ points (1.6 SD). The comparable gains for the placebo group were 0.5 DQ points and 5.1 DQ points respectively. At the end of the 4 month trial, these children had similar developmental levels to those who were not iron deficient in the first place. It is worth pausing to reflect quite how large the effect of iron supplementation is in this age group. Effects sizes of 0.1 SD or 0.2 SD are considered large in the field of education. Effect sizes of more than 1 SD are very rare, but were found for both cognitive and motor developments in this study. This illustrates a key argument for health and nutrition programmes presented in Chapter 1: improving children's health and nutrition brings substantial benefits for cognitive development and education.

A number of other studies have conducted supplementation trials over a similar time period (>=12 weeks), although none had the same rigorous experimental design. One other study in Indonesia succeeded in eliminating developmental differences between iron deficient and iron replete children after supplementation, while in two other studies, in Chile[47] and Costa Rica[4], there was no observed effect of supplementation. However, in the Costa Rica study, children whose iron status recovered completely also showed improvement in their mental and psychomotor development indices. A number of short-term trials (<15 days) have also been conducted. There is no evidence of improvement of iron deficient children in such trials[46].

Taken together, the evidence from all trials suggests that iron supplementation can improve the development of children under 2 years of age if sustained over a sufficiently long period of time (~12 weeks). However, this conclusion is based largely on the results of one trial.

Iron deficiency also affects mental development in children aged 2 to 6 years

As with infants, iron deficiency leads to cognitive impairments in preschool children. The first set of studies in this age group look at the association between iron deficiency anaemia and cognitive function. A number of such studies have compared iron deficient anaemic children with iron replete children. In Guatemala, children with iron deficiency anaemia took longer to learn a discrimination task than their iron replete peers[50]. The difference between the two groups was substantial in this test (>3 SD), although there were no differences in two other tests. Similarly, Indonesian children with iron deficiency anaemia were slower than iron replete children in a categorisation task[51], although the two groups performed similarly on tests of learning and vocabulary; no such differences were found with younger children in one study in India[52].

Does iron deficiency anaemia cause cognitive impairments? Can iron supplementation improve cognitive function? These questions are answered in our second set of studies in the preschool age group. All five studies answer yes to both questions. All five have found improvements in the cognitive function of iron deficient children following iron supplementation, including improvements in a learning task[50,51] and in an IQ test[52, Studies 1 and 2]. One study in Zanzibar[53] gave 12 months of iron supplementation and deworming treatment to children aged 6 to 59 months from a population in which iron deficiency was common. They found that iron supplementation improved preschoolers' language and motor outcomes by 0.14 SD and 0.18 SD respectively.

The conclusion from studies of preschool children and infants is that iron deficiency can have a substantial effect on children's cognitive development. The next section considers the implications this has for children's later development in the school-age years and beyond.

Iron deficient infants have poor cognitive abilities in adolescence

Several effects of iron deficiency in infancy indicate that resulting cognitive impairments may be long term. Irreversible changes to the developing brain can result in permanent impairment of cognitive function. Also, because the behaviour of anaemic infants and their caregivers is different from that of healthy infants, the amount of stimulation children receive will also differ. This is likely to affect their cognitive development.

A number of studies have investigated the long-term effects of iron deficiency[46]. The most comprehensive of these followed a group of Costa Rican infants for more than 10 years[54,55]. At 12 to 24 months of age, 30 of the group of 191 infants had moderate anaemia and received treatment. At age 5 years, formerly anaemic infants performed more poorly on a range of tests of motor function and non-verbal intelligence after accounting for differences between the two groups in a number of variables such as socioeconomic status, birth weight, maternal IQ, height and education. Verbal skills were more equally matched between groups. At age 11 to 12 years, the formerly anaemic group performed more poorly in writing and arithmetic, on a motor test and on a test of spatial memory. Only the older children were poorer in a selective attention test. The formerly anaemic group were more likely to have a number of behavioural problems. They were more anxious and depressed, had more attention problems, social problems and overall behavioural problems. They were also more likely to repeat grades at school and to be referred to special education services.

Similar findings have emerged from a number of other studies. Anaemic infants in Chile[56] were later found to have lower IQs and poorer performance on a range of tests of motor, verbal and visual abilities at 5 years of age. There is a clear continuity between impaired cognitive development and poor academic achievement for children with anaemia. A study with infants in Israel[57] found that a difference in haemoglobin (Hb) levels of 1g/l at 9 months (10.5g/l vs. 11.5g/l) was associated with a reduction of 1.75 IQ points at 5 years of age (although no effect on developmental levels was found at 2 and 3 years of age). Children in the anaemic group were found to be less task-oriented than control children and were lagging behind in educational achievement (by 0.7 SD) in second grade[58].

All of the above studies followed a relatively small group of children from infancy in order to chart their development. One study in the United States took a different approach[59] by retrospectively linking educational assessments of 10 year old children with data on their nutritional status between birth and 5 years. They found that children with low levels of haemoglobin in early childhood were more likely to be classified has having mild to moderate mental retardation at age 10. (A decrease of 1g/l of Hb was associated with being 1.28 times more likely to be classed as having mental retardation.)

It should be noted that none of the studies reported in this section allow causal inferences to be drawn. In each study, the anaemic group most likely differed from the control groups on a number of background variables such as socioeconomic status. One study[56] found that in comparison to the control group, the homes of anaemic infants were less stimulating and their mothers were more depressed and less affectionate. Thus, we cannot be sure that differences in performance between groups are not attributable to these other background characteristics, even though comprehensive attempts were made to control for them statistically in most studies.

Nevertheless, the evidence of the effect of anaemia and iron deficiency on the brain, on the behaviours of infants, preschoolers and their caregivers and the suggestion that the effect is a long-term one, combine to make a persuasive case for early intervention to prevent iron deficiency.

Other nutritional deficiencies

Iodine deficiency during pregnancy causes long-term cognitive impairment

Iodine is required for the synthesis of thyroid hormones. These hormones, in turn, are required for brain development, which occurs during fetal and early postnatal life[60]. Mental development is affected by both maternal hypothyroidism (a deficiency in production of the thyroid hormone by mothers), which affects development of the fetal brain during the third trimester, and hypothyroidism in the newborn which affects postnatal brain development[61]. In either case, a spectrum of neurological disorder can ensue, from severe mental retardation associated with cretinism (see Chapter 3) to more subtle neurological impairments. Nearly 50 million people suffer from iodine deficiency related brain damage. A relatively small proportion of these (<10 per cent) are cretins with the remainder suffering more mild impairments.

Iodine supplementation in pregnancy reduces cretinism and improves IQ and school achievement between 8 and 15 years of age in one study[62] and between 14 and 16 years of age in another[63].

The clear evidence from these intervention studies is supported by findings of impaired cognitive function in adults and children living in iodine deficient areas. An estimate based on an analysis of 21 studies suggests that general intelligence is 0.40 SD lower in iodine deficient areas[64]. However, there is no clear evidence for the cognitive benefits of targeting preschool children with iodine supplementation.

Zinc supplementation can improve cognitive abilities

Few other micronutrients have been studied in relation to their effect on the cognitive development of young children but there is a growing body of literature on zinc and mental development. In the UK, children with dyslexia were found to be deficient in zinc and to have higher concentrations of toxic metals in their sweat and hair[65]. Animal studies show that zinc deficiency in offspring causes impaired learning which can be corrected by zinc supplementation[66].

One study has been conducted to investigate the impact of maternal zinc supplementation on cognitive development. This study in Bangladesh[67,68] gave zinc (30mg daily) or a placebo (cellulose) to pregnant women from 4 months gestation to delivery. At 6 months, the children whose mothers had been given zinc supplementation had poorer outcomes in both mental development and psychomotor development indices. This is likely due to an imbalance of micronutrients and suggests caution should be exercised when targeting single micronutrient deficiencies for supplementation.

Summary: Micronutrient deficiencies and child development

Iron deficiency anaemia

- Iron has many functions in the brain. This is evident in slower neural conduction recorded in infants with iron deficiency.
- Infants with iron deficiency anaemia are more easily tired, less attentive, show less delight and playfulness and maintain closer contact with caregivers.
- Sustained (>12 weeks) supplementation of iron deficient infants can improve developmental scores substantially (>1 SD).
- In the preschool age group, iron supplementation leads consistently to improved cognitive function among iron deficient children.
- Compared with healthy controls, iron deficient infants have poor educational achievement and more behavioural problems later in life.

Other nutritional deficiencies

- Iodine supplementation in pregnancy has long-term impacts on IQ and school achievement.
- Zinc supplementation improves the development of undernourished infants. The improvement is accentuated with additional psychosocial stimulation. Maternal zinc supplementation in isolation can impair cognitive development of infants.

A more recent study in Jamaica assessed the impact of zinc supplementation and psychosocial stimulation on the development of undernourished infants and young children aged 9 to 30 months[69]. This study was a randomised controlled trial with four study groups receiving zinc supplementation, psychosocial stimulation, both, or neither intervention. Stimulation consisted of weekly home visits to demonstrate play activities and to encourage mother-child interaction. After 6 months, the overall Development Quotient (measured on the Griffiths Mental Development Scales) was modestly improved in the group receiving psychosocial stimulation (2.5 DQ points, or 0.17 SD) but no overall improvement was seen in the group receiving zinc alone. An analysis of sub-scales of the Griffiths Mental Development Scales showed that psychosocial stimulation improved hearing and speech (7.3 DQ points, 0.49 SD) and performance (6.0 DQ points, 0.4 SD) sub-scales and zinc supplementation improved hand and eye coordination (4.4 DQ points, 0.29 SD). The greatest benefits were seen for the group who received both interventions. Overall the development quotient was improved by an additional 5.2 DQ points (0.35 SD) in this group. Performance on the hand and eye coordination sub-scale was improved by an additional 10.1 DQ points (0.67 SD). This study demonstrates that, in contrast with the results of the Bangladesh study, supplementation with zinc, in isolation, can be beneficial to children's mental development. Furthermore, the study underscores the importance of combining psychosocial and nutritional interventions in this age group.

Infectious disease and child development

Malaria infection has long-term effects on education

A number of diseases directly affect the central nervous system. Of these, the most common in low income countries is cerebral malaria. In the previous chapters we saw that cerebral malaria is a leading cause of deaths among children under 5 years and that, of those who survive, a significant proportion suffer neurological problems which effectively prevent them from attending school in many areas of the world. Many other children suffer more subtle cognitive deficits which may affect their ability to learn later on in life. In Kenya, children aged 6 to 7 years were studied 3 to 4 years after hospitalisation due to cerebral malaria with impaired consciousness[70] and were found to be 4.5 times more likely than other children from similar backgrounds to suffer cognitive impairment ranging from severe learning difficulties requiring care, to mild cognitive impairments. Almost half of such children had had no neurological problems at the time of hospitalisation. Similarly, in Senegal children aged 5 to 12 years were found to have impaired cognitive abilities due to a bout of cerebral malaria with coma before the age of 5. The primary cognitive deficit was likely to have been to children's attention[2]. A third study in the Gambia looked at children who suffered from cerebral malaria that was not accompanied by neurological symptoms at the time[71]. These children had poorer balance 3.4 years after recovery implying some impaired motor development. However, no other cognitive deficit was found.

In such studies, the likelihood is that cognitive impairments are a direct result of the episode of cerebral malaria. In addition to the immediate effects, a bout of cerebral malaria can leave an individual with an increased chance of epileptic episodes which in turn can lead to cognitive impairment[72].

Cerebral malaria is clearly a major cause of cognitive impairment in preschool children. However, the incidence of serious attacks of malaria declines sharply in the school years. Is there evidence that early childhood malaria continues to be a problem for children's learning? Only one study has investigated the long-term impact of early childhood malaria prevention on subsequent cognitive development. This study in the Gambia[73] found that children who were protected from malaria for three consecutive transmission seasons before the age of 5 years had improved cognitive performance at age 17 to 21 years. For those who had received the longest protection from malaria, the improvement in cognitive function was around 0.4 SD.

There was also clear evidence of the impact of malaria protection on educational attainment. Children who had been protected from malaria in early childhood stayed at school for around one additional year (see Figure 4.3).

Other behavioural problems have been associated with cerebral malaria. Psychotic episodes have been reported following bouts of cerebral malaria in Nigeria[74,75]. Thus, there are multiple ways in which cerebral malaria can affect behaviour.

Another indirect pathway by which children can be affected by malaria is as a result of malaria infection during pregnancy. Pregnant women are twice as likely as non-pregnant women to be bitten by mosquitoes[76], increasing their vulnerability to malaria infection. This increases the likelihood of stillbirth. If children survive they have an increased chance of having low birth weight. As demonstrated earlier in this chapter, low birth weight is associated with a long-term impairment in cognitive development.

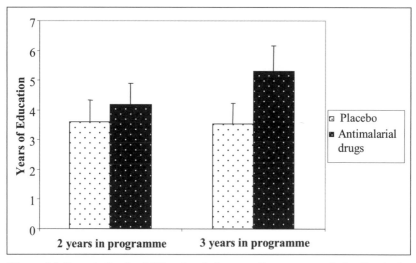

Figure 4.3. Impact of early childhood malaria prevention on years of schooling in the Gambia. *Source:* Jukes *et al.* (2006)[73].

Worm infections may affect the cognitive abilities of preschoolers

There is good evidence that worm infections affect children's ability to learn in the school-age years (see Chapter 5). It is likely that worm infections have a similar impact for preschool children. Infections are prevalent in this age group although worm loads typically do not reach peak intensity until the school-age years. A study in Kenya showed that 28 per cent of preschool children (6 months to 5 years) harboured hookworm infection, 76 per cent were anaemic and that anaemia was more severe in those children with hookworm[77]. Evidence of a cognitive impact of worm infections in preschoolers is not clear. Two studies[78,79] have demonstrated cognitive improvements in preschool children following combined treatment for worm infections and iron deficiency anaemia. However, neither study was able to disentangle the effects of the two treatments.

Infants with Giardia infection have lower IQ at age 9

The final parasitic infection considered in this section is *Giardia lamblia*. Giardia is a protozoan parasite that is ingested and inhabits the gastrointestinal tract. It contributes significantly to caseloads of diarrhoea. One study in Peru[80] followed a cohort of children, some of whom had had diarrhoeal diseases, parasitic infection and severe malnutrition in the first 2 years of life. Severe malnutrition at this age was associated with an IQ 10 points (0.67 SD) lower at age 9 years. Those who had suffered two or more episodes of giardiasis per year scored 4.1 IQ points (0.27 SD) lower than children with one episode or fewer per year. It is likely that this association is due to Giardia infection causing, or acting as an index of, malnutrition.

Otitis media (Glue Ear) affects language development of poor children

Otitis media is an inflammation of the middle ear cavity often resulting from spread of infection from the nose or throat. In acute cases, pus is produced, pressurising the eardrum and causing perforation in chronic cases.

Otitis media is common in rich and poor countries[81]. Around 6 per cent of primary school and pre-primary school children were found to have chronic otitis media with effusion (OME) in Vietnam[82] and South India[83]. In Tanzania, 9.4 per cent of rural and 1.4 per cent of urban schoolchildren were found to have chronic otitis media with effusion.

OME has mild effects on language development[84] and other cognitive skills. The effect depends on the length of infection and caregiver environment[85]. Children from low socioeconomic backgrounds are more likely to suffer effects of OME. This result suggests that the effects of OME may be greater in poor countries than in rich countries, although research is yet to be carried out to demonstrate this.

Survivors of meningitis perform poorly at school

The previous chapter discussed the high prevalence of meningitis in poor countries, the associated mortality and the risk of severe neurological problems for survivors. Other survivors of meningitis do not have obvious neurological problems and yet suffer long-term behavioural problems.

In Ghana, survivors of a meningitis epidemic, from a wide range of ages (2 to 73 years), were more likely to suffer from feelings of tiredness (OR=1.47) and were more often reported by relatives to have insomnia (OR=2.31)[86]. However, meningitis infection did not affect school attendance among school-age cases.

Studies in rich countries have found that children who appear well after bacterial meningitis have more non-specific symptoms like headache, and more signs and symptoms indicating inattention, hyperactivity and impulsiveness than their siblings[87]. Survivors of bacterial or viral meningitis go on to perform more poorly at school, to be more likely to repeat a grade and to be referred to a special needs school. They are also more likely to have behavioural problems in the home[88]. Cognitive abilities are also affected. Survivors of meningitis have lower IQs than their peers (~0.3 SD) at ages 7 and 12 years[89] with no signs of the gap narrowing with age. Conversely, behavioural problems of meningitis survivors are greater than their peers and actually increase with age.

Summary: Infectious disease and child development

- Protecting children from malaria in early childhood has a long-term impact on cognitive abilities and can increase educational attainment by around one grade (i.e. an extra year in school).
- There is suggestive evidence that deworming preschoolers can improve their cognitive abilities.
- Infection with *Giardia lamblia* parasites is associated with cognitive impairment in the long term.
- Otitis media with effusion (glue ear) can lead to impaired language development.
- Survivors of meningitis have poorer cognitive abilities and poorer performance at school.

Interventions: What works?

Table 4.1 summarises the impact of health interventions on cognitive development in early childhood. Only studies giving quality evidence from experimental interventions are included. Such evidence is available for four types of intervention: iron supplementation, iron supplementation plus deworming, psychosocial stimulation of malnourished children and nutritional supplementation. Most interventions are aimed at a specific target group (iron deficient or malnourished children) although two interventions are aimed at all children in a community.

The first striking point about the table is that all studies have demonstrated a positive impact. Note, this table is not a selective account of health interventions that have worked; rather it is a summary of all experimental interventions found in the literature. In contrast with interventions in other age groups, it is notable that a positive impact on at least one cognitive test was found in every case. The size of the impacts are also worthy of note. Where the size of the impact is quantified, all interventions aimed at nutritionally disadvantaged groups improve cognitive abilities by at least two-thirds of a standard deviation. In the context of the literature on improving cognitive abilities these are remarkably large effects, equivalent to an increase of 10 IQ points or lifting a child from the 25th percentile to the 50th percentile of the ability distribution. The two studies that showed modest effects were targeted at a community cohort rather than a nutritionally disadvantaged population.

Table 4.2 shows the studies which have followed up preschool health interventions and assessed their cognitive impact in the long-term. Three of the studies tracked participants to adolescence and found that improvements in cognitive function persisted. Both studies in Jamaica found sizeable long-term effects of psychosocial but no effects of nutritional supplementation. The malaria prevention study in the Gambia is of interest because relatively large impacts were found even though the intervention was provided for a whole community rather than just for sick children. All four studies show that the early cognitive benefits of preschool health interventions carry through to benefit children's education in the long term.

Conclusion

Extensive research has been conducted on the educational effects of early childhood health and nutrition interventions. The breadth and depth of this research allows for a number of general conclusions to be drawn relating to four of our arguments to support health and nutrition programmes.

Disease affects education throughout childhood

This chapter presented the first half of a two-part argument that primary school education is affected by the health and nutrition of children at all ages. Two points emerge from the current chapter that relate to this argument. First, children's cognitive abilities and educational achievement at primary school are affected by conditions they suffered long before entering primary school. In this chapter we saw how young children with undernutrition, iron deficiency anaemia, iodine deficiency, malaria, or parasites causing diarrhoeal diseases have impaired cognitive abilities later on in life, when they are learning at school. So,

Table 4.1. Impact of health interventions on cognitive development during early childhood.

Study	Country	Intervention	Age (months/years)	Sample characteristics	Effect size (SD)	Outcomes
Jukes et al. in prep[79]	India	Iron (30 day) + deworming	2-6	ECD pupils	0.18	Attention
Seshadri & Golpadas 1989 study 1[52]	India	Iron (60 day)	5-8	Anaemic vs. non-anaemic	+ve	IQ
Seshadri & Golpadas 1989 study 2[52]	India	Iron (60 day)	5-6	Anaemic vs. non-anaemic boys	0.33 / 0.67	Verbal IQ / Performance IQ
Soewondo 1989[51]	Indonesia	Iron (56 day)	4	Anaemic vs. non-anaemic	+ve / No effect	Learning task / 3 cognitive tests
Stoltzfus 2001[53]	Zanzibar	12 months iron + deworming	6-59 months	Community	0.14	Language
McKay 1978[22]	Colombia	Nutrition + education from 42 months	84 months	Malnourished	0.80	Cognitive ability
Grantham-McGregor 1991[23]	Jamaica	Psychosocial stimulation	9-24 months	Malnourished	0.79	Mental development
Grantham-McGregor 1991[23]	Jamaica	Nutritional supplementation	9-24 months	Malnourished	0.66	Mental development
Vermeersch & Kremer 2004[20]	Kenya	School feeding	4-6	ECD pupils	0.4[1]	Educational achievement

[1]Effect only for pupils of most experienced teachers.

Table 4.2. Long-term impact of health interventions in early childhood on cognitive and educational outcomes.

Study	Country	Intervention	Age (years)	Sample characteristics	Effect size (SD)	Outcomes
Grantham-McGregor et al. 1994[25]	Jamaica	Stimulation	14	Severely malnourished	0.68	IQ
Walker et al. 2000[27]	Jamaica	Stimulation	11-12	Stunted	0.38	IQ
Walker et al. 2000[27]	Jamaica	Nutritional supplements	11-12	Stunted	No effect	IQ
Chang et al. 2002[28]	Jamaica	Stimulation/ Nutritional supplements	11-12	Stunted	No effect	Education tests
Pollitt et al. 1997[30]	Indonesia	Nutritional supplements	8	Initially >18 months	+ve	Working memory
Jukes et al. 2006[73]	Gambia	Malaria prevention	14-19	Community cohort	0.25-0.4	Cognitive function

school performance is not affected only by school-age health and nutrition. The second point is that health and nutrition interventions appear to be effective at all ages. There is no evidence that interventions early in life are most effective and that programmes targeting older preschool children are too late to benefit their development. This is an argument that will be developed in the next chapter when we consider children of school-age.

Improving children's health and nutrition brings substantial benefits for cognitive development and education

It is quite remarkable how consistently health and nutrition programmes are shown to bring substantial benefits to cognitive development in this age group. Every intervention study reported has found a benefit for development with effect sizes as large as 0.7 SD to 0.8 SD in several cases. The best evidence of educational benefits is found for feeding programmes, iron supplementation and malaria prevention.

Improving health and nutrition brings the greatest educational benefits to the poor and most vulnerable

Most of the programmes reported in this chapter were provided to poor communities. The consistently large educational effects found are testament to the substantial benefits improved health and nutrition can bring to the poor. In addition, there were several examples of programmes that benefit the most vulnerable to the greatest extent. We saw how nutritional supplements led to the greatest cognitive improvements in young girls in Colombia, and the children from the poorest families in Guatemala. We saw how the cognitive abilities of low birth weight babies benefited more from breast-feeding than other children and how malaria prevention in the Gambia led to a reduction in the enrolment gap between boys and girls.

Health and education reinforce one another

Work in the preschool age group provides many examples of how health and education work together. In some cases, health and nutrition interventions increase the potential for cognitive growth but are not effective unless accompanied by educational interventions to exploit this potential. In Guatemala, nutritional supplementation improved achievement only for the children who stayed in school the longest. In Vietnam, a combination of nutritional supplementation and an early childhood education programme was required to reverse cognitive delays of undernourished children. In Jamaica, psychosocial stimulation has been effectively combined with nutritional supplements and with zinc supplements to improve development. In Kenya, school feeding was effective only for schools with experienced teachers. Health and education clearly do reinforce each other. The converse is also true. Poor health impairs development only where children lack sufficient mental stimulation. In Brazil, cognitive delays were seen for low birth weight babies only if they received little stimulation at home.

These four arguments for health and nutrition programmes are well supported by evidence from infants and preschool children. In the next chapter, these same four aspects of health and nutrition programmes will be the focus. We will see how school health and nutrition programmes also benefit the most vulnerable to the greatest extent and help reinforce the benefits of education. In doing so, we will complete the picture of health and nutrition and its effects on education throughout childhood.

Chapter 5

Health, nutrition and educational achievement of school-age children

The previous chapter demonstrated that as children enter school they may already be suffering from the cognitive disadvantages of growing up with health and nutrition problems. That is, even children who are currently in good health may lag behind peers in school work because they were ill or nutritionally compromised during infancy or the preschool years at important times for cognitive or social development.

We now consider the additional effects on children's education due to continuing – or newly acquired – infections and nutritional deficiencies during the school-age years. The distinction between the current and previous chapters is made largely on the basis of programmatic considerations. The aim is to determine the approach to treating and preventing conditions of ill health and poor nutrition which yields the highest dividends in terms of children's education. Are some conditions most effectively addressed during critical periods of children's cognitive, language or social development? If this opportunity is missed during the preschool years can children's education still be improved by interventions taking place in the school-age years? Or is it more important, in any case, to ensure that children are healthy and well nourished while they are actually in the process of studying? These are some of the questions that motivate the review of research in this chapter.

To pre-empt the answers to these questions, we argue that targeting school-age children's health and nutrition is indeed an effective way to improve their education. Indeed, such programmes are the focus of this book because of this effectiveness. The case for school health and nutrition programmes rests on the fact that disease affects education throughout childhood. This is one of the four arguments for health and nutrition programmes discussed in the previous

 ©CAB International 2008. *School Health, Nutrition and Education for All: Levelling the Playing Field* (M.C.H. Jukes *et al.*)

chapter. The other three are also reiterated in the current chapter: improving children's health and nutrition brings substantial benefits for cognitive development and education; improving health and nutrition brings the greatest educational benefits to the poor and most vulnerable; and health and education reinforce one another. We will look at how these arguments apply to school health and nutrition programmes in two parts: nutritional deficiencies and their effect on education followed by infectious disease and their effect on education.

Nutritional deficiencies in school-age children

School-age children are affected by many of the same nutritional problems – chronic undernutrition and micronutrient deficiencies – that initiate long-term cognitive delays in preschoolers. These will be considered later on in this section. First we look at a condition specific to this chapter – one that doesn't necessarily cause long-term impairments but has a big impact on children's ability to learn in school: hunger.

Hungry children have poor cognitive abilities

Short-term hunger is a condition we all experience and one that is easy to induce for the purpose of studying its cognitive effects. Consequently, the effects of this condition are quite well understood. Work at Cardiff University in the UK has established that missing breakfast impairs performance of adults on short-term memory tasks throughout the morning. By contrast, reaction times are improved by caffeine intake but not by eating breakfast[1]. Similar cognitive profiles for the effect of missing breakfast have been found for children in low income countries[2] but in this context the effect is dependent on the long-term nutritional status of the children. A number of studies[2-4] have found that missing breakfast impairs performance to a greater extent for children of poor nutritional status. In one study in Jamaica, eating breakfast improved scores of malnourished children by 0.25 SD more than adequately nourished children in three cognitive tests of memory and speed of processing and one test of arithmetic (see Figure 5.1)[3]. This finding echoes those from several different sections of this book that the effects of various health and nutritional problems on children's education interact with one another. Invariably the children who are worst off to begin with are those that suffer the most.

Short-term hunger has a number of other effects that may affect school performance indirectly. General mood deteriorates[1] and stress increases[5] with hunger in adults. Observations in Jamaican schools[6] suggested that providing children with breakfast had another effect on behaviour with an intriguing dependence on school quality. In better organised schools, children were more likely to concentrate when they had eaten breakfast. In poorly organised schools, children who had eaten breakfast talked more and were less attentive to school work. In other words, school feeding appeared to energise behaviour; school quality determined the purpose to which this extra energy was directed. This is another example of how health and education reinforce one another and suggests that children benefit most from a simultaneous improvement in nutrition and school quality.

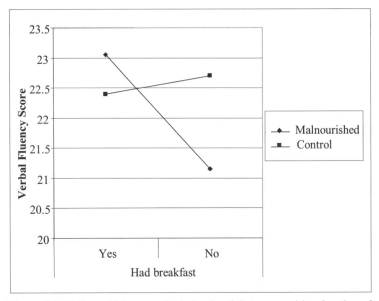

Figure 5.1. Differential impact of missing breakfast on cognitive function of malnourished and well nourished children in Jamaica. *Source:* Simeon (1989)[3].

The evidence discussed so far suggests that school feeding has the potential to confer benefits to children's education through two mechanisms – improved cognitive function due to the alleviation of short-term hunger (discussed above) and improved school attendance (discussed in Chapter 3). Before considering the evidence for such programmes, let us look at a third mechanism – improved nutritional status.

Undernourished children perform poorly at school

The previous section showed that going without food can affect children's school performance in the short term, but what of chronic undernutrition? Going without adequate food for an extended period of time affects physical growth. But how does undernutrition affect mental growth? A commonly used measure of chronic undernutrition is height-for-age. This measures the number of standard deviations above or below the mean height of a healthy population of children at the same age. It is a common finding that children with low height-for-age perform poorly at school[7,8]. Two studies have found that 1 SD increase in height-for-age is associated with an increase of 0.1 SD in tests of arithmetic[9,10] and language[10]. However, it is difficult to infer that undernutrition is the cause of poor school performance given that factors such as poverty tend to be correlated with both nutritional status and scholastic achievement[11] (see Box 4.3 in the previous chapter).

The link between chronic undernutrition and school performance receives further support from two studies which have found specific patterns of behaviour and cognitive performance associated with nutritional status. In Kenya, better nourished children scored more highly on tests of verbal comprehension and a test of non-verbal reasoning (the Raven's Progressive Matrices Test). Girls who were better nourished were also more attentive during class[12]. A similar study in Egypt found gender-specific patterns of behaviour related to nutritional indices. Better nourished boys had improved classroom behaviour and increased activity levels; better nourished girls had a higher verbal ability and were more involved in class[13].

Although these results are suggestive of a link between chronic undernutrition and school performance, evidence is needed from long-term supplementation trials. Several such studies have been conducted with younger children and were discussed in the previous chapter. One of these studies bridged the preschool and school-age years. Working with chronically undernourished children in Colombian families of low socioeconomic status in the year before entering school, McKay[14] found that a programme of nutritional supplementation, health care and education was able to narrow the gap in cognitive abilities between programme participants and wealthier peers. This suggests that undernourished school-age children are likely to have poorer cognitive abilities and that there are programmatic possibilities for improving these abilities. The main such programmatic option for school-age children is the school feeding programme.

School feeding programmes have modest effects on educational achievement

Two trials have been conducted with school-age children. One study in Jamaica[15] gave breakfast to children for a year and found that the scores in arithmetic improved by 0.11 SD for the youngest children (in Grade 2 at the beginning of the study). Analyses suggested that this improvement was because children attended school more frequently and because they studied more effectively while at school[4]. The feeding programme did not improve arithmetic in older children or reading and spelling in children of any age. In Kenya, schoolchildren were given milk, meat or energy supplements for 21 months[16], with the three types of supplements containing the same number of calories. Children who were given meat improved their arithmetic scores by 0.15 SD and their performance on the Raven's Progressive Matrices Test (a test of non-verbal reasoning) by 0.16 SD but did not improve on verbal comprehension. Of these three tests, only arithmetic scores were improved by the energy supplements (by 0.11 SD) while the milk supplement had no effect on children's test scores. Meat differs from other supplements (such as milk) by providing available zinc and iron. Such micronutrients have an impact on cognitive abilities (see below and Chapter 4) and their presence may explain the relative effectiveness of meat supplements in improving test scores. The relative benefits of one supplement over another should not detract from the overall finding that school feeding programmes have a small impact on cognitive abilities compared to other types of interventions. This is a small return for the expense (see Chapter 6) of providing a daily meal for children for a year or more. It may be that the main benefit of school feeding programmes is to encourage children to attend school (see Chapter 3).

Iron supplementation improves cognitive function of school-age children

There is good evidence that iron deficiency anaemia (IDA) affects children's cognitive abilities[17]. In the previous chapter we saw how young children with iron deficiency have impaired development, and are less active than healthy children. If anaemic children are entering school with such impairments their performance at school is likely to suffer. Indeed, in Thailand children with anaemia and/or iron deficiency are substantially delayed (~2-3 SD) in tests of language and of general reasoning ability, although not in arithmetic scores. Similarly there were substantial, albeit smaller differences (~1 SD) between Indonesian schoolchildren with IDA and iron replete children in their performance on a range of school exams[18], although the children did not differ in a test of concentration.

Such studies are suggestive of the problems that children with IDA may face at school. However, as with other observation studies discussed in this text, they cannot demonstrate that IDA causes cognitive impairment. Evidence for the link between iron deficiency anaemia and cognitive function is strengthened by findings that 2 to 3 months of daily iron supplementation is effective in improving cognitive abilities. In school-age children, iron supplementation improves performance on tests of memory and visual/motor coordination,[19, Studies 3 and 4] in concentration and school exam performance[18]. In many of these cases the improvement in performance is large (~0.5 SD) but in others, iron supplementation does not completely eliminate differences in cognitive performance and educational achievement even when differences in iron status are eliminated. Indeed, one study[20] found no improvement in school achievement in response to iron therapy. If iron deficiency does impair children's learning, it is likely that a short course of supplementation is insufficient to remedy the problem. Concentration may recover fairly quickly in response to treatment but it may take a sustained period of improved concentration before children catch up on years of lost learning.

Cognitive development is delayed in iodine deficient areas

Schoolchildren living in iodine deficient areas have poorer cognitive abilities[21-23] than children living in iodine sufficient areas. In the interests of designing control strategies it is important to know whether this represents the concurrent effect of iodine deficiency on schoolchildren's cognitive function and educational achievement or whether it represents the long-term effect of severe iodine deficiency in early childhood (see Chapter 3).

Some evidence addresses this issue and questions the long-term nature of this effect and the severity of the iodine deficiency which causes it. Work with schoolchildren in Bangladesh[24] found that general cognitive abilities and mathematics test scores were related to indicators of *recent* iodine deficiency, as opposed to a chronic deficiency. Other work suggests that it is not only severe iodine deficiency that affects mental functioning. Schoolchildren in Benin with only mild iodine deficiency were found to have poorer hearing which was in turn associated with poorer mental abilities[25]. Thus, it is possible that iodine deficiency in the school-age years holds back educational achievement.

However, these studies are not conclusive and stronger evidence is required from randomised controlled trials. A number of such have been conducted in recent years with little clear evidence that iodine supplementation improves mental function. Iodine deficient children in Bangladesh did not show improvements in cognitive and motor performance after 4 months of supplementation with iodised poppy seed oil, even though the treatment improved their iodine status[26]. By contrast, in Benin it was found that schoolchildren whose iodine status improved the most after supplementation with iodised poppy seed oil also showed the greatest improvement in cognitive performance[27]. Unfortunately, complications in the study design made it difficult to conclude that the improvements in cognitive performance were a result of the iodine supplementation.

It is difficult to say for certain whether iodine deficiency continues to affect cognitive performance in the school-age years. More supplementation trials, both preventive and remedial, could resolve this issue. As it stands, there is insufficient evidence to recommend iodine supplementation as a means of improving the mental abilities and educational achievement of schoolchildren.

Multiple micronutrients improve cognitive abilities

Given the frequent overlap and clustering of micronutrient deficiencies, multiple micronutrient supplementation or fortified foods may be a cost-effective strategy to address nutrient deficiencies in school-age children, in addition to synergistic effects between certain micronutrients.

Three studies have analysed the effect of multiple micronutrients on cognitive abilities. In China, 6 to 9 year olds' cognitive function was improved to a greater extent by a combination of zinc supplements and multiple micronutrients over a period of 10 weeks, than by either intervention alone[28]. In KwaZulu-Natal, children receiving biscuits fortified with iron, iodine and beta-carotene (a precursor of vitamin A) for 43 weeks had improved short-term memory in comparison to control children[29]. However, performance on eight other tests did not improve.

Similar results were found in India[30]. A year long course of multiple micronutrient supplementation improved the attention of school-age children but not their performance on two other cognitive tests, or on tests of IQ or educational achievement. These mixed results suggest that multiple micronutrient supplementation is a promising area of research but it is too early to say whether it is more beneficial than individual supplementation, for example with iron, in its effect on cognitive function.

Summary: Nutrition in school-age children

- Hungry children have impaired cognitive abilities, especially if they are chronically undernourished.
- Poorly nourished children are less attentive in class.
- School feeding programmes have a modest effect on educational achievement.
- Iron deficient children perform poorly at school but iron supplementation improves their cognitive function.
- Cognitive development is delayed in iodine deficient areas; iodine supplementation has not proved to be a successful intervention in school-age children.
- Multiple micronutrient supplementation can improve cognitive abilities and is a promising school health and nutrition intervention.

Infectious disease in school-age children

The second half of this chapter looks at infectious disease. As discussed in Chapter 2, worm infections are a particularly significant infectious disease in the school-age years. But malaria, colds and flu, and HIV&AIDS (directly and indirectly) also affect children's learning in this age group.

Deworming improves the potential to learn

Severe and chronic infection with parasitic helminths during children's development may have consequences for their cognitive performance and ultimately their educational achievement. These effects on cognitive function may occur as a result of one or a combination of symptoms associated with infection. For example, one of the main consequences of infection with many species of helminth is iron deficiency[31] and there is much evidence that iron deficiency anaemia is associated with impaired cognitive performance and development (see above and Chapter 4). Also, helminth infection can result in poorer growth rates[31] and this may also be a route by which infection leads to impaired performance because undernutrition is associated with cognitive development and educational achievement[8,32].

Evidence suggests that schoolchildren do suffer such cognitive effects of worm infections. In South America, Africa and Asia, schoolchildren who are infected with worms are found to perform poorly in tests of cognitive function[33]. This is particularly true for children who are infected with multiple species of helminths or with heavy loads of helminths. In this way, studies of worm infections support one of the reasons for school health programmes discussed in Chapter 1: poor health and nutrition has the biggest educational impact on the most vulnerable children. An example of this comes from a study in Tanzania[34] which found that a heavy infection with schistosomiasis delayed reaction time only for children who were also undernourished. These children are likely to benefit the most from any deworming treatment.

These findings could be the result of confounding factors such as poverty or nutrition (see Box 4.3 for a discussion of confounding factors). However, it appears such factors do not account for the relationship between worm infection and cognitive function as far as it is possible for us to measure and account for poverty and nutritional status[34]. Such studies support the case that worm infections genuinely cause poor cognitive function.

However, when infected children are given deworming treatment, immediate educational and cognitive benefits are not always apparent. On the one hand, benefits are clear in some cases. One study in Jamaica[35] found around a 0.2 SD increase in three memory tests after treatment for infection with whipworm (*Trichuris trichiura*). Children in this study had moderate to heavy infections with this worm (i.e. children with light infections were excluded). On the other hand, several studies have failed to improve the learning of all children through treatment[35-38]. Some children did benefit from these deworming programmes, however. Improvements in cognitive abilities or education were found for younger children[35], children with poor nutritional status[36] or with the heaviest worm loads[36]. This restriction of benefits to sub-groups of children illustrates two important points. First, as with so many interventions discussed in this book, the biggest impact is found for the most vulnerable children – the youngest, the most heavily infected and the malnourished. Second, the success of deworming as an educational intervention depends on the characteristics of the population. When considering the value of a deworming programme it is important to have good information about the worm loads and levels of malnutrition in the area.

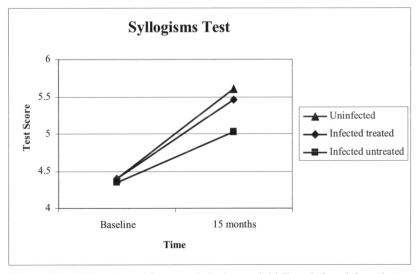

Figure 5.2. Children treated for worm infections or initially uninfected, learn better on how to perform a syllogisms test over time, than children who continue to be infected. *Source:* Grigorenko *et al.* (2006)[39].

For most children, treatment alone cannot eradicate the cumulative effects of lifelong infection nor compensate for years of missed learning opportunities. Deworming does not lead inevitably to improved cognitive development but it does provide children with the potential to learn. Children in Tanzania who were given deworming treatment did not improve their performance in various cognitive tests but did benefit more from a teaching session in which they were shown how to perform the tests[39]. Performance on a reasoning task at the end of the study was around 0.25 SD higher in treated children than in those who still carried worm infections. The treated children's performance was similar to children who began the study without infection. This suggests that children are more ready to learn after treatment for worm infections and that they may be able to catch up with uninfected peers if this learning potential is exploited effectively in the classroom (see Figure 5.2).

The likely implication of this evidence for the design of programmes is that preventing uninfected children from becoming infected is the most effective way of seeing educational benefits. For children who are already infected, treatment may improve their educational outcomes in the long term; but short-term benefits are not possible by deworming alone.

School-based malaria prevention improves educational achievement

A number of recent studies have assessed the impact of school-based malaria prevention on cognitive function and educational achievement. A randomised controlled trial in Sri Lanka[40] gave regular treatment with chloroquine or a placebo to children in Grades 1 to 4 of primary school. Children receiving chloroquine scored 0.65 SD higher in a mathematics test and 0.59 SD higher in a test of language. Improved scores were partly attributable to reduced absenteeism. Children in this study attended school around 5 days per year longer as a result of the intervention (see Chapter 3). Another recent study[41] used a different approach to preventing anaemia in schoolchildren. Following successful use of intermittent preventive treatment (IPT) with infants and pregnant women this approach to malaria control was evaluated with schoolchildren in Kenya. Children were given 2 doses of antimalarials each year. This resulted in a large (55 per cent) reduction in the prevalence of anaemia in these children. The subsequent effect on children's cognitive abilities was also substantial. Children protected from malaria performed better in two tests of sustained attention (by 1.09 SD and 0.92 SD) than children given a placebo.

Although evidence is still accumulating on the best approach to malaria prevention in schools, this type of intervention clearly has great potential to benefit children's education. Malaria prevention produces some of the largest improvements in cognitive abilities and educational achievement seen in this age group.

Colds delay reactions; flu impairs attention

The effect of colds and flu on cognitive function is better understood than for most conditions. Unlike with other diseases scientists have been able to experimentally infect adult participants with influenza and with the common cold, allowing a much clearer understanding of their effects[42]. In one study, subjects infected with the influenza virus responded more slowly to tasks requiring them to detect stimuli appearing at irregular intervals, probably due to the effect of infection on attention functions. The effect was substantial: the reaction time increased by 57 per cent. This is significantly greater than with other regularly occurring effects on cognitive function, such as performing tasks in the middle of the night or after alcohol consumption, which typically increase reaction time by around 10 per cent. In fact, even sub-clinical infections increase reaction time significantly. This is one more example of how common illnesses can be surprisingly debilitating to specific cognitive functions.

The effect of influenza infections appears to be confined to the attention function, however. Infection has no effect on hand-eye coordination tasks, simple motor tasks, reaction time tasks not involving attention, nor on working memory and reasoning tasks.

Experimentally induced cold infections have a similarly specific effect but on different cognitive functions. With colds, it is the hand-eye coordination that is primarily affected and attention functions are spared. Sub-clinical infections also affect performance and the effects of a cold on cognitive function may persist after primary symptoms have disappeared.

The effect of colds on memory function shows an interesting pattern. Recall of several words or digits is unaffected by colds as is the recall of information learned before the onset of the cold. However, colds affect the ability to follow a story and recall relevant information subsequently. Infected individuals tend to focus on irrelevant information in the story and are unable to recall more important themes from the story. Although this result and all others reported in this section have been conducted with adults, the implication for children and their performance in the classroom is clear. If colds have similar effects in children as in adults they are likely to target specific skills such as the processing and storage of new complex information – precisely those skills needed to learn in the classroom.

Colds can also amplify or moderate the effect of other factors on performance, such as caffeine and noise levels. This highlights a common theme in research on the effects of disease and poor nutrition on cognitive function – various conditions are likely to interact with others and the study of conditions in isolation, especially those that typically co-occur, may not be relevant to the conditions as they occur naturally.

Programmatic implications of these findings are not clear. Work has yet to be carried out to investigate the educational benefits of preventing cold and flu infections in schools.

Children with HIV infection perform poorly at school

HIV&AIDS differs from other diseases discussed in this chapter in that almost all affected school-age children are infected via vertical transmission. That is, they have been infected with the HIV virus since birth. Therefore, with HIV&AIDS it is not possible to distinguish between the long-term effects of infection in infancy (the focus of Chapter 4) and the concurrent effects of infection in the school-age child (the focus of the current chapter). However, it is worth emphasising that research in high income countries has demonstrated that school-age children with HIV infections are found to have lower IQ and academic achievement, language[43] and visual motor functioning[44]. This is certainly due in part to the effects of HIV on cognitive development before

Summary: Infection in school-age children

- Deworming can improve learning when combined with an education intervention. Otherwise deworming improves cognitive ability for children with the heaviest infections or with poor nutrition.
- School-based malaria programmes bring substantial benefits to educational achievement.
- Colds delay reactions and flu impairs attention, but the programmatic response to these problems is not clear.
- Children with HIV perform poorly at school but antiretroviral therapy improves cognitive abilities and daily living skills.

children enrol in school, but it is encouraging for programmatic responses to HIV that such deficits in cognitive function can be reduced or reversed with antiretroviral therapy[45-47]. Although a wide age range of children took part in these studies, spanning preschool and the school-age years, it seems likely that therapy directed specifically at school-age children will also be beneficial. One study[48] found that improvement in cognitive abilities in response to 36 months of antiretroviral therapy was greater for children older than 6 years compared with younger children. The benefits for schooling of antiretroviral therapy are not confined to improvements in cognitive function. A number of studies have found that the adaptive behaviour (skills required for everyday activities) of children living with HIV improves after treatment[46, 49-51].

Antiretroviral therapy then can bring direct benefits to children's education as well as indirect benefits by improving the health of parents and helping to avoid the tragedy of children becoming orphans, discussed in the next section.

Orphanhood leads to psychosocial problems in school-age children

HIV&AIDS brings with it many other factors that may affect children's education. Children living with HIV&AIDS are more likely than other children to have lost one or both parents. Evidence suggests that children living with HIV&AIDS suffer from psychosocial problems. One study in Tanzania has found increased rates of depression in AIDS orphans[52]. A more recent study in Zimbabwe[53] found that orphans had a higher rating on a measure of depression than non-orphans by 0.13 SD for boys and 0.20 SD for girls. Female orphans were also more likely to suffer from poor self-esteem.

Although these studies did not consider the educational consequences of psychosocial problems, there is reason to believe that school performance will suffer from parental HIV&AIDS, through the additional demands on children, particularly girls, to care for their sick parents, and through the psychosocial impact discussed above. At the same time, attending school can help mitigate the impact of orphanhood on children's mental health[54].

Interventions: What works?

Table 5.1 summarises findings from trials assessing the impact of school health and nutrition interventions on cognitive abilities and/or educational achievement. There is good evidence for five types of interventions. Iron supplementation and malaria prevention have the largest effects. School feeding has a smaller effect even when sustained over a whole year. Deworming can have an impact on learning, especially when combined with an educational intervention. Otherwise the biggest impacts are found for younger children or children with heavy infections or who are malnourished. The first trials of multiple micronutrient supplementation in schoolchildren show improvements in test scores.

The overview of cognitive effects in Table 5.1 should be considered together with evidence of improvements in school attendance discussed in Chapter 3. It is interesting that the two interventions with equivocal evidence of cognitive improvements (deworming and feeding) are those interventions that show the strongest effects on school attendance. Thus, all five interventions listed in the tables, show clear educational benefits of some kind. The missing pieces of information in the overall pictures of intervention effectiveness are the costs of these interventions. These are considered in the next chapter. First, we pause to reflect on the themes emerging from evidence in this chapter.

Conclusion

Studies of school-age children discussed in this chapter complete the body of evidence presented in Chapters 3 and 4 which support four central themes concerning the educational impact of health and nutrition programmes.

Disease affects education throughout childhood

Evidence from school-age children helps develop the argument that poor health and nutrition affect education throughout childhood. In doing so, it argues for the need to provide programmes to school-age children as well as to preschool children. The previous chapter presented the case for early interventions, preventing cognitive damage before it can be done. The present chapter shows that there is continued potential for intervention in the school-age years to help children's education while they are in the process of studying. This is because many of the health and nutrition interventions discussed in this chapter show substantial benefits for children's education.

Table 5.1. Impact of health interventions on cognitive function and educational achievement of school-age children.

Study	Country	Intervention	Age (years)	Sample characteristics	Effect size (SD)	Outcomes
Iron Pollitt et al. 1989[20]	Thailand	Iron supplementation	9-11	Iron deficient	No effect No effect	Raven's Progressive Matrices Education tests
Soemantri et al. 1985[18]	Indonesia	Iron supplementation	10-11	Iron deficient	0.42 0.51	Education tests Concentration
Seshadri & Golpadas 1989 (studies 3&4)[19]	India	Iron supplementation	8-15	Iron deficient	+ve[1]	4 cognitive tests
Feeding Powell et al. 1998[15]	Jamaica	Daily breakfast for 1 year	M= 9		0.11[2] No effect No effect	Arithmetic Reading Spelling
Whaley et al. 2003[16]	Kenya	Meat/energy[3] supplement for 2 years	M=7.6		0.16[4] No effect 0.11 – 0.15	Raven's Progressive Matrices Verbal comp Arithmetic
Micronutrients Vazir et al.2006[30]	India	Multiple micronutrients for 1 year	6-15		+ve No effect No effect No effect	Attention test 2 cognitive tests IQ 4 education tests

[1] Effect is positive in: 2/4 cognitive tests for girls given 60mg of iron daily and boys given 30mg of iron, and all tests for boys given 40mg of iron. [2]Effect only for youngest children. [3]A milk supplement had no effect. [4]No effect of energy supplement.

Table 5.1. *continued.* Impact of health interventions on cognitive function and educational achievement of school-age children.

Study	Country	Intervention	Age (years)	Sample characteristics	Effect size (SD)	Outcomes
Malaria Prevention Fernando et al. 2006[40]	Sri Lanka	Antimalaria pills (chloroquine)	6-12		0.65	Mathematics
					0.59	Language
Clarke et al. in prep[41]	Kenya	IPT (amodiaquine and sulfadoxine-pyrimethamine)	10-18		0.92-1.09	Sustained attention
Deworming Nokes et al. 1992[55]	Jamaica	Deworming	9-12	Moderate-high whipworm infection	0.16-0.26	3 cognitive tests
					No effect	5 cognitive tests
Simeon et al. 1995[36]	Jamaica		7-10	Mild-moderate whipworm	~0.15[5]	Verbal fluency
					No effect	6 cognitive tests
Simeon et al. 1995[37]	Jamaica		6-12	Whipworm infection	0.16[6]	Spelling
					No effect	Reading
					No effect	Arithmetic
Sternberg et al. 1997[38]	Jamaica		M=10.3	Mild-moderate whipworm	No effect	7 cognitive tests
Nokes et al. 1999[35]	China	Deworming	5-16	S. japonicum infection	0.59[7]	Verbal fluency
					Ns	4 cognitive tests
Grigorenko et al. 2006[39]	Tanzania	Deworming	11-13	Heavy S. haematobium	0.08-0.32	3 'dynamic' cognitive tests
				Moderate hookworm infection	0.09	1 cognitive tests
					No effect	7 cognitive tests

[5]Effect only for children with poor nutritional status. [6]Effect only for children with heaviest worm loads. [7]Effect only for youngest children.

Improving children's health and nutrition brings substantial benefits for cognitive development and education

Table 5.1 summarised the size of educational benefits found for school health and nutrition interventions. The largest effects are found for iron supplementation and malaria prevention with deworming, school feeding programmes and micronutrient supplementation also having sizeable impacts. The effect sizes are not as large as for preschool children but they are still substantial in comparison with many other education interventions. In the next chapter, we argue that school health and nutrition programmes are inexpensive, sustainable and their goals (to improve education) are clearly tied to those of the schools in which they operate. These factors allow school health and nutrition programmes to bring these sizeable benefits to children's learning, year after year.

Improving health and nutrition brings the greatest educational benefits to the poor and most vulnerable

The poor and disadvantaged benefit the most from school health and nutrition interventions as much as from interventions targeted at younger children discussed in Chapter 4. In this chapter we saw how the biggest educational benefits of deworming were seen for children with poor nutritional status or with the heaviest worm loads. Conversely, missing breakfast reduces cognitive abilities to the greatest extent for children who are already chronically undernourished.

The poor suffer the Double Jeopardy of being more likely to be affected by poor health and nutrition and of being more likely to have cognitive delays or educational problems as a result. Because of this, school health and nutrition programmes have the potential to benefit the poorest to the greatest extent and thus, to promote equity. In the next two chapters, we look at another feature of these programmes which helps to promote equity – they are very effective at reaching poor and marginalised communities.

Health and education reinforce one another

The current chapter also supported findings from programmes in early childhood and infancy that education and health reinforce each other. In this chapter we saw how a deworming programme in Tanzania did not benefit educational achievement of children but it did improve their ability to learn a new task that was taught to them. In Jamaica, a school feeding programme only benefited children attending well ordered schools. Both of these findings suggest that school health and nutrition programmes will be most effective in improving education when combined with other improvements in education quality.

These conclusions complete the picture presented of why health and nutrition programmes are so effective in improving education and equity. As we have argued, these reasons to support health and nutrition programmes, apply equally to infants, preschool children and school-age children. In the final two chapters, we will pay particular attention to the benefits for delivering health and nutrition programmes through schools, namely that such programmes are cost-effective and reach the neediest children.

Chapter 6

Costs and benefits of school health and nutrition interventions

In the previous chapters we developed the argument for health and nutrition programmes based on the current state of health and nutrition in young children (Chapter 2) and its effect on education (Chapters 3 to 5). Many of these arguments applied equally to infants, preschoolers and school-age children. The current chapter shifts the focus to school-age children and presents a major reason why health and nutrition programmes can be delivered successfully through schools: improving health and nutrition through schools is highly cost-effective.

The argument for cost-effectiveness is developed in several steps. In the first step we show that health and nutrition interventions are cheaper when delivered through schools (the 'cost' half of the 'cost-effectiveness' argument). The second step is to show that such interventions are effective in improving children's health. In fact, school health and nutrition interventions have a large impact on children's health given how little they cost and are thus considered highly cost-effective compared with other health interventions. The third step in the argument is to consider the impact of these programmes on children's education. We have argued throughout the book that health and nutrition interventions are effective at improving children's education. Yet, typical cost-effectiveness estimates have been restricted to improvements in health and have ignored the educational benefits. In this chapter we consider ways to calculate the cost-effectiveness of school health and nutrition programmes as a means to improve children's education. In the final sections of this chapter we show that school health and nutrition programmes are more cost-effective than other educational interventions and we estimate the potential global impact of school health and nutrition interventions if expanded to all areas where children suffer from poor health and nutrition.

Intervention costs and cost-effectiveness

Delivery costs of school health and nutrition programmes are low

A key issue in addressing the costs of the new approach to school health and nutrition programmes is the significant savings offered by using the school system, rather than the health system infrastructure as the key delivery mechanism. This provides a pre-existing mechanism, so costs are at the margins, but also a system which aims to be sustainable and pervasive, to reach marginalised children and to promote social equity. Table 6.1 shows the cost of providing deworming treatment to schoolchildren through different delivery mechanisms[1]. In the 1980s and early 1990s most programmes were 'vertical' in nature and involved a mobile health team which visited communities giving treatment to everyone or just to those infected. The cost of delivering these drugs ranged from 21 to 51 cents. Note that this is just the cost of delivering the treatment and does not include the price of the drug itself. By contrast, the cost of delivering school-based programmes is as little as 3 to 4 cents. This is more than ten times less expensive than the most costly mobile treatment teams.

Annual costs of providing some other common school-based interventions to students are given in Table 6.2. This table illustrates two important points. First, that some of the most widely needed interventions can be provided at remarkably low cost. Second, that there is significant diversity in the costs of interventions, and that this must be borne in mind when identifying a school health package.

Table 6.1. Examples of delivery costs for a single mass treatment.

Strategy	Drug	Country	Delivery cost per treatment	
			US$	Percentage of total cost (%)
Mobile team to community	Albendazole	Montserrat	0.51	67
	Albendazole	Bangladesh	n/a	42
	Levamisole	Nigeria	0.32	81
	Praziquantel	Tanzania	0.21	24
School-based	Albendazole	Ghana	0.04	17
	Albendazole	Tanzania	0.03	13
Out-of-school children		Egypt	0.16-0.21	40-47

Source: Guyatt (2003)[1].

Table 6.2. Annual per capita costs of school-based health and nutrition interventions delivered by teachers.

Condition	Intervention	Cost US$
Intestinal worms	Albendazole or mebendazole	0.03-0.20
Schistosomiasis	Praziquantel	0.20-0.71
Vitamin A deficiency	Vitamin A supplementation	0.04
Iodine deficiency	Iodine supplementation	0.30-0.40
Iron deficiency and anaemia	Iron folate supplementation	0.10
Refractive errors of vision	Spectacles	2.50-3.50
Clinically diagnosed conditions	Physical examination	11.5
Undernutrition, hunger	School feeding	21.6-151.2 21.26-84.5[*]

[*]For South America and Africa, costs are standardised for 1,000 kcal for 180 days.
Source: Del Rosso (1999)[2], Partnership for Child Development (1999)[3].

Cost-effectiveness of school health and nutrition programmes for improving children's health

The cost-effectiveness of interventions can be assessed in terms of the cost per DALY (disability adjusted life year) gained. DALYs reflects the total amount of healthy life lost to a disease, whether from premature mortality or from some degree of disability during a lifetime. Using this measure Table 6.3 shows that school health and nutrition programmes are relatively cost-effective compared with other public health interventions.

Table 6.3. The cost per DALY gained by school health and nutrition programmes relative to other common public health interventions.

Health Intervention	Cost per DALY gained
Expanded Programme on Immunisation Plus	12-30
School Health and Nutrition Programmes	20-34
Family Planning Services	20-150
Integrated Management of Childhood Illness	30-100
Prenatal and Delivery Care	30-100
Tobacco and Alcohol Prevention Programmes	35-55

Source: Bobadilla *et al.* (1994)[4].

This table is concerned only with improvements in children's health but the benefits of school health and nutrition programmes extend beyond physical health. We have argued that improved education is also a major benefit. In the following sections we consider the cost-effectiveness of school health and nutrition programmes for improving children's education.

Cost-effectiveness of school health and nutrition programmes for improving education

The impact of various conditions of poor health and nutrition is typically expressed as "Global Burden of Disease Estimates"[5], which focus on mortality and physical morbidity attributable to diseases. In these estimates, schoolchildren are often perceived as healthy if they are not suffering from any clear physical symptoms of a disease. Prevalent chronic conditions with insidious effects are often invisible in public health statistics and as a result, the apparent benefits of school health and nutrition programmes are underestimated. The measures of mortality or health-related disability used do not capture the impact of ill health on cognitive development or on educational outcome effects that are of particular relevance at an age when the foundations are laid for lifelong learning and for productivity in adulthood.

Including education in burden of disease estimates is difficult because simple metrics have not been developed to quantify the lifelong impact on children's learning. For health outcomes, the concept of disability adjusted life years (DALYs) has proved valuable. This measure calculates the number of years of life lost by premature death due to a disease but also estimates the equivalent fraction of a year lost through suffering an illness. In these estimates, being severely ill for a year may be considered equivalent to losing, say, 6 months of that year to premature death. The advantage of such a method is that it allows one to estimate and quantify the total impact of a disease over a lifetime. We need an equivalent measure for the impact of improved education throughout people's lives.

One way to calculate the lifelong benefits of education is to consider its impact on economic productivity. This has the advantage of quantifying the effect in a way that can be compared with other interventions and gives us a way of summing the effect over a lifetime. The most common approach to assessing the economic benefits of education has been to calculate the increase in wages resulting from an increase in years of education.

Economic benefits of increased school participation

Evidence suggests that an additional year spent at school increases productivity. Increased years of schooling is associated with higher worker productivity in waged employment and in other economically productive activities such as farming[6-8]. The impact of education on productivity is quantified in calculations of rates of return to education. The rates of return to education can be thought of as the percentage increase in annual wage resulting from an additional year spent at school. Overall, studies find that the returns to years of schooling in wages are higher in poor countries than in rich countries. For sub-Saharan Africa, they find a 12 per cent rate of return to one additional year in school, compared to 10 per cent for Asian countries, 7.5 per cent for OECD countries, 12 per cent for Latin America and the Caribbean. These returns are very high, even allowing for a portion of this return to years of schooling to be based on ability and other factors rather, that are not the product of schooling itself[9].

How do school health and nutrition interventions lead to wage increases? Where improved health results in children spending more time at school we can make use of the rates of returns calculations discussed above to estimate the benefits of interventions. For example, in Chapter 3, we discussed a study in Kenya that found deworming treatment improved primary school participation by 9.3 per cent with an estimated 0.14 additional years of education per pupil treated[10] over the course of their schooling. The study used information on rates of return to education in Kenya, to estimate that treating one child increased lifetime wages by US$30[a] at a cost of only US$0.49 for the deworming treatment. This investment seems a little more costly when you consider that additional teacher resources may be needed to cope with increased attendance. Even taking this into account the benefit of US$30 can be gained from an investment of under US$10. This is a high return on a small investment.

This example illustrates how cost-effective school health and nutrition interventions can be. However, the method used to calculate the economic benefits cannot be easily applied to other evidence presented in this book. We have argued that much of the benefit of improved health and nutrition comes in the form of improved cognitive abilities or educational achievement. How do these outcomes affect lifetime earnings? One problem we have in answering this question is that most of the evidence presented in the previous chapters was relatively short term. For example, we know how children's learning improves for the year or two following a deworming programme but can we work out if children are likely to leave school with higher education attainment and achievement as a result of this programme? We will try and address this issue by thinking about the long-term impact of improved health and nutrition, first on cognitive abilities and then on educational attainment. Our starting point is to summarise the short-term impact of school health and nutrition programmes. Table 6.4 shows the improvement in cognitive and educational tests following selected school health and nutrition interventions. The impact of interventions varies in the range of 0.25 SD and 0.4 SD and is illustrative of the typical range of benefit for such interventions outlined in Table 5.1 in the previous chapter.

---

[a] The figure of US$30 reflects the fact that people value future earnings less than current earnings. (A bird in the hand is worth two in the bush.) Future earnings are 'discounted to the present' in the jargon.

We will use these typical values as the basis for calculating the long-term impact on cognitive abilities and educational attainment in the next section.

Economic benefits of long-term improvements in cognitive abilities

The increase in cognitive abilities shown in Table 6.4 could diminish with time. Alternatively it could lead to greater educational opportunities (see below) and cognitive abilities could increase further with time. If we take the middle ground and assume that the short-term benefits are roughly maintained over the course of schooling, that they result in long-term benefits of a similar size, then the cognitive abilities of children when they leave school will be improved by around 0.25 SD.

So how do these improved abilities translate into improved earnings? In the United States[11], an increase in IQ of one standard deviation is associated with an increase in wages of over 11 per cent. Similar estimates have been made for the relationship between cognitive abilities and wages in Ghana, Kenya, Pakistan, South Africa and Tanzania[12]. The estimated increase in wages associated with a standard deviation increase in cognitive abilities ranges from 5 to 48 per cent, with typical values around 20 per cent. Extrapolating this result, a 0.25 SD increase in cognitive abilities which is a reasonable estimate of the benefit resulting from a school health and nutrition intervention, would lead to around a 5 per cent increase in wages. For most of the countries listed above (excluding South Africa) this represents around a US$25 increase in yearly earnings due to a school health and nutrition intervention[b].

Improved cognition leads to improved educational attainment

Another way to think about the long-term benefits of improved cognitive abilities is to assess their implications for increased educational attainment – often synonymous with the number of years spent at school. The relationship between improved cognitive abilities and years of schooling can be estimated in a number of ways. One approach is to consider improvements in cognitive abilities and educational achievement in the early years of schooling and to estimate the long-term impact they may have on time spent at school. In countries where many children drop out before they finish primary school, how well they do in school can be influential. If children perform poorly in the early years of schooling they may quickly become discouraged and drop-out. Conversely, a small improvement in achievement in the early grades may be

---

[b] This is based on gross national income per capita which ranges from US$400 to US$700 in these countries, with a median around US$500. Thus, US$500 x 5% = US$25.

Table 6.4. Cognitive impact of selected school health and nutrition interventions.

Study	Intervention & duration	Age	Sample characteristics	Effect size (SD)	Outcomes
Simeon & Grantham-McGregor 1989[13]	Breakfast (1 day)	9-10	Malnourished	0.25	Memory, speed of processing, arithmetic
Soemantri et al. 1985[14]	Iron supplementation (2 months)	10-11	Iron deficient	0.4	Education
Nokes et al. 1992[15]	Deworming (3 months)	9-12	Moderate/heavy whipworm	0.25	Memory
Grigorenko et al. 2006[16]	Deworming (18 months)	11-13	Heavy hookworm/bilharzia	0.25	Learning

enough to ensure promotion to the next grade level and renewed motivation and ability to succeed. In this way, a small improvement in scores in the early years can have a large cumulative impact in the long term.

One study in South Africa[17] assessed the direct impact of test scores in Grade 2 on progression through primary school. They found that children who score 0.25 SD above the average in Grade 2 exams were around 1.5 times as likely to complete Grade 7[c]. Figure 6.1 shows how the pattern of drop-out is different for children who scored 0.25 SD higher than the mean in their Grade 2 exams. If a school health and nutrition intervention raised exams scores by 0.25 SD and had a similar impact on drop-out rates, the extra cumulative years of schooling averages at 1.19 years per pupil over the course of primary school years.

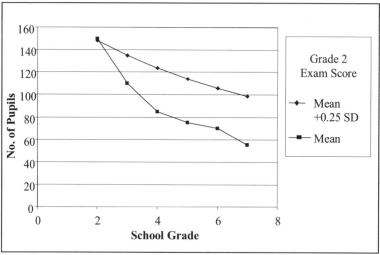

Figure 6.1. Estimating school drop-out with and without school health and nutrition interventions, after Liddell and Rae (2001)[17].

Such calculations involve many assumptions and are likely to overestimate the impact of health and nutrition programmes on children's educational attainment. For this reason it is important to pursue other methods for estimating this effect. The relationship between lower achievement and years of schooling can be estimated indirectly by considering the number of years of schooling required for sick children to catch up with healthy children. For example, in Tanzania[18] heavy schistosomiasis infection was associated with a decrease in arithmetic scores of 1.4 marks (0.25 SD). An extra year's schooling was associated with an increase in arithmetic scores of 2.2 marks (0.42 SD). Thus,

---

[c] Authors' calculations based on reported results from Liddell and Rae (2001).

the negative effect of a heavy schistosomiasis infection was equivalent to that of missing just over half a year's schooling.

The cognitive gains from an extra year of schooling can also be estimated retrospectively. In a study of adults in South Africa[19], each additional year of primary schooling was associated with a more modest 0.1 SD increase in cognitive test scores. According to these estimates, a typical increase of 0.25 SD associated with a school health and nutrition intervention is equivalent to an additional 2.5 years of schooling.

We have presented three different methods for estimating the effect of school health and nutrition interventions on educational attainment. We estimate that these interventions would increase educational attainment by between 6 months and 2.5 years. That is, children would stay at school for between half a year and two and a half years longer as a result of a school health and nutrition intervention. This estimate is consistent with observations from the field[20]. A recent study in the Gambia found that preventing malaria in early childhood led to children staying on at school for around one year longer. This result helps us to think about the impact of school health and nutrition interventions on economic productivity after school. An additional year of primary schooling leads to around a 10 per cent increase in wages in poor countries. For the countries discussed in the previous section (Ghana, Kenya, Pakistan and Tanzania) this would represent an increase in wages of around US$50 a year. The cost–benefit analysis is more complex in this case, however. The additional year of schooling comes with additional costs. So we cannot view the increase in wages of US$50 a year as the return solely on the small investment in improved health. But we know that an additional year of primary school is a very good investment in poor countries. In this situation, improved health can be seen as the catalyst – the facilitating factor that makes the investment in education possible.

In conclusion, the estimates presented in this section are necessarily speculative. However, they serve to illustrate that investing in school health and nutrition interventions can cost less than US$1 per child, but the improvements in education that result lead to economic returns many times the value of the investment.

The global impact of school health and nutrition programmes

So far, our discussion in this chapter has focused on the individual. But, a key argument for school health and nutrition programmes presented in Chapter 1, and developed in Chapter 2, is that diseases affecting education are highly prevalent. Thus, school health and nutrition programmes have the potential to bring the benefits discussed above to vast numbers of children. We now try and quantify this potential global impact.

An approach to estimating the global burden of disease in terms of cognition is illustrated by Table 6.5. The table examines three common diseases in terms of their impact on the cognitive ability of the estimated 562 million school-age children in poor countries[21]. Deficits in test scores attributable to these diseases are converted into an equivalent loss in IQ points. Clearly, conditions of poor health and nutrition have more complex effects on cognitive functioning than this conversion into IQ points implies. However, IQ provides a widely understood scale on which to illustrate the global impact of cognitive impairments resulting from disease.

Table 6.5. Estimates of the global cognitive impact of common diseases of school-age children in poor countries.

Common diseases	Prevalence (%)	Total cases (millions)	IQ points lost per child	Additional cases of IQ <70 (millions)	Lost years of schooling (millions)
Worms	30	169	3.75	15.8	201
Stunting	52	292	3	21.6	284
Anaemia	53	298	6	45.6	524

Table 6.5 estimates the additional number of cases of children with IQ <70 (part of the definition of mild mental retardation)[22] attributable to each disease. The table also estimates the lost years of schooling attributable to impaired cognitive function. These estimates are based on the relationship between cognitive function and educational attainment illustrated in Figure 6.1 and on the calculations discussed in the text accompanying this figure.

The estimates in Table 6.5 suggests that three common diseases may result in an additional 15 and 45 million cases of mild mental retardation in primary school children, and a loss of the equivalent of between 200 million and 524 million years of primary schooling worldwide. While the precision of these striking figures may be open to debate, they clearly show that even minor cognitive deficits resulting from ubiquitous diseases can result in an extraordinarily large scale of effect.

Comparative cost-effectiveness of school health and nutrition programmes

The educational gains from school health and nutrition programmes should be considered in the context of alternative educational inputs, such as improving teacher salaries and qualifications, reducing class size, improving school facility infrastructure, and providing instructional materials. There are many studies that relate student outcomes to school characteristics, but few of these provide information on the relative or actual costs of the educational inputs[23]. The costs are, however, likely to be substantially greater than for the school health and nutrition interventions considered here. Despite these higher costs, the evidence from the few randomised evaluations that have been conducted, suggests that the scale of impact of additional education inputs, is typically of a similar or lower magnitude compared with school health and nutrition programmes[24]. In Brazil and India instructional materials (such as additional textbooks) had the highest productivity, raising student test scores significantly more than other inputs for each dollar spent. However even these interventions only have an impact of between 0.06 SD and 0.4 SD[25]. In Kenya, textbook provision had no impact on the lowest achieving 60 per cent of the students, and raised test scores by 0.2 SD for the highest achieving 40 per cent of the students. Relating these results to the findings in the previous section and to the annual per pupil costs, school health and nutrition interventions appear very cost-effective compared with the highest productivity inputs. They improve educational achievement by a similar amount (0.25-0.4 SD) at a much lower cost.

Similar conclusions can be drawn from interventions to increase school attendance. In Kenya, deworming led to increased school attendance at the cost of US$3.50 per additional year at school. The equivalent costs for other programmes were US$36 for school feeding and US$99 for subsidised school uniforms. Recently, conditional cash transfer programmes have been viewed as potentially very cost-effective methods to increase school enrolment[26]. These programmes are generally large in scope, representing a commitment of between 0.1 per cent and 0.2 per cent of gross national income. The PROGRESA programme (an education, health and nutrition programme) in Mexico is estimated to have increased enrolment by 3.4 per cent and increased schooling by 0.66 years, with an average cash transfer (for Grades 3 to 8) of about US$136 per child per school year. Gains from a similar programme in Nicaragua were estimated at 0.45 years of school at a cost of US$77 per year. Comparing these results with those presented for school health and nutrition programmes, in both cases the conditional cash transfer approach is apparently at the lower end of effectiveness and at the higher end of cost. Thus, it appears that school health and nutrition interventions are very cost-effective.

From cost-effectiveness to programme design

When designing a programme, effectiveness and cost-effectiveness are key considerations. However, there may be many dimensions to costs. Identifying the appropriate mix of interventions for a given circumstance can be facilitated by a decision matrix that incorporates these multiple dimensions. Box 6.1 illustrates how the government of Eritrea set about prioritising interventions in the Eritrea school health and nutrition programme. In the next chapter we consider how such programmes are designed and implemented.

**Box 6.1. The Eritrea school health and nutrition programme:
How to identify priority interventions**

1. The first step taken in developing the strategic plan was to review the different health conditions affecting schoolchildren in Eritrea and to consider how these can be addressed using the four components of the FRESH framework. This enabled the identification of conditions affecting Eritrean children that could effectively be addressed through school-based health and nutrition services.

2. Once conditions that could be addressed through school-based health and nutrition services had been identified, decision-making matrices were constructed to enable the need, benefit, cost and feasibility of different services to be considered (see Tables A and B below).

3. The results of the Situation Analysis and the knowledge and experience of members of the Ministries of Health and Education were then used to determine which health services needed to be delivered in different parts of the country.

Table A: Decision-making matrix for conditions which can be treated by teachers in schools.

Condition	Need†	Scale of benefit		Cost (US$ per capita)	Feasibility of universal access‡
		Education	Health		
Bilharzia	+++*	+++	+++	0.80	+++
Anaemia	+++*	+++	+++	1.20	+++
Vitamin A supplementation	+++	+	+++	0.30	+++
Skin infections	+	+	+	3.00	++
First aid	++	++	++	0.50	++

Table B: Decision-making matrix for conditions where teachers can refer children to local health services.

Condition	Need†	Scale of benefit		Cost (US$ per capita)	Feasibility of universal access‡
		Education	Health		
Dental caries	++	+	+++	30.00	+
Refractive error	+++	+++	++	5.00	++
Eye infections	+++	++	+++	3.00	++
Hearing impairment	++	+++	+	200.00	+
Ear infections	++	+++	+++	3.00	++
Malnutrition	++	+++	+++	30.00	++

Where +++= high, ++= moderate, += low; *In certain areas.
†Evidence from Situation Analysis & MoH experience. ‡Experience elsewhere.

Conclusion

School health and nutrition interventions are highly cost-effective

In this chapter we have argued that a major reason to implement school health and nutrition interventions is that they are highly cost-effective. Their low cost results from the advantages to using educational infrastructure to deliver interventions. Their effectiveness has been considered mainly in terms of the impact they have on children's health. In this regard, school health and nutrition interventions are indeed cost-effective. But this overlooks the lifelong impact on children's education. We have estimated this impact in the current chapter. School health and nutrition interventions are highly cost-effective in this regard also. The economic benefits of the school health and nutrition interventions resulting from improved education exceed their cost several times over. They are also cheaper than many other education interventions that produce a similar impact on children's learning.

School health and nutrition interventions can have a massive global impact

In previous chapters we discussed how improved health and nutrition has a large impact on education and how the diseases of poor health and nutrition are very prevalent. In the current chapter we have brought these two findings together to estimate the global impact of these diseases on education. The number of years of schooling lost annually to diseases such as anaemia may be more than 500 million. By tackling such problems, school health and nutrition interventions can have a massive positive impact on education around the world. The next chapter considers how such programmes can be implemented.

Chapter 7

School health and nutrition programmes

In this final chapter we discuss another way in which school health and nutrition programmes level the playing field. We have already presented evidence that school health and nutrition interventions promote equity because the poor bear the greatest burden of disease and because these diseases have the biggest educational impact on the poor. In this chapter we see how the delivery of these interventions can also be pro-poor. School health and nutrition programmes delivered through schools are sustainable and reach the poorest children. We go on to look at the policy options for implementing such programmes and the frameworks that guide their design.

The previous chapters have shown that ill health and malnutrition are common among schoolchildren in low income countries, and have a significant impact on education participation and achievement. The evidence indicates that the presence of these conditions at school-age reflects both experiences in early childhood, and experiences at school-age. Ensuring good health at school-age therefore requires a "life cycle" approach to intervention, starting *in utero* and continuing throughout child development. In programmatic terms this implies a sequence of programmes to promote maternal and reproductive health, management of childhood illness, early child care and development and school health and nutrition. All these elements are required if a school-age child is to be healthy and well nourished, and to take full advantage of the opportunity for education.

This book focuses on the health, nutrition and education of the school-age child, and on the programmes that can be implemented at school-age to promote positive outcomes. Information on the essential "upstream" interventions, such as Integrated Management of Childhood Illness (IMCI) and Early Child Development (ECD) is available elsewhere[1,2].

 ©CAB International 2008. *School Health, Nutrition and Education for All: Levelling the Playing Field (*M.C.H. Jukes *et al.)*

There has been a significant shift in focus of school health and nutrition programmes in low income countries over the last two decades. The programmes have moved away from a medical approach that favoured elite schools in urban centres, and towards a focus on improving health and nutrition for all children, particularly the poor and disadvantaged. This change began in the 1980s when research started to confirm that good health and nutrition were strongly related to educational achievement. These research findings led to the recognition that school health and nutrition programmes were not only important contributors to health outcomes, but were also essential elements of efforts to improve education access and completion, particularly for the poor. In the 1990s, when the concept of Education for All (EFA) was first launched, school health and nutrition programmes were adopted by the education sector, and began to be incorporated within EFA programmes. The success of these initial efforts led to demand from countries and agencies for a more coordinated and systematic approach to programming.

Policy and economic issues in designing interventions

Poverty is a key consideration in the design of school health and nutrition programmes. The negative correlation between ill health and malnutrition and income level is clearly demonstrated both in cross-country comparisons and within countries[3], partly because lower incomes and higher poverty themselves promote disease and inadequate diet. Similarly, children who are not enrolled in school come from households with lower income levels[4]. Furthermore, evidence presented in previous chapters demonstrates that the educational impact of disease and poor nutrition is greatest for the poorest children. These factors suggest that there will be a greater return to school health services that are pro-poor and specifically linked to efforts to achieve EFA. Thus, expanded coverage is a critical factor for the effectiveness of school health and nutrition programmes.

Coverage has been limited for historical reasons. Many school health programmes, particularly in Africa, have descended from colonial antecedents that were intended to serve the minority of children that had access to school in urban centres or elite boarding facilities. They rely on specific infrastructures and services – such as health team school visits, school nurses and in-school clinics – that are additional to the normal range of health service provision, and are beyond the means of most low income countries to make available universally. An analysis of a school nurse programme in KwaZulu-Natal, for example, showed that despite a relatively high investment (the cost per student targeted was US$11.5), the coverage was inadequate (18 per cent) and almost no cases of ill health detected resulted in effective referral and treatment[5].

The case for overcoming such barriers to coverage is strong. Traditional medical practice emphasises treatment after individual diagnosis. But analysis of the types of health interventions that are part of more inclusive school health and nutrition programmes, such as deworming and micronutrient supplements, suggests that mass approaches are preferable, on technical, economic and equity grounds, to approaches that require diagnostic screening[6]. Furthermore, we might argue, on the grounds of equity, in favour of avoiding the need for access to health service facilities. This is because access to health services is positively and significantly associated with income. Poorer populations (which experience more ill health) would be systemically overlooked by intervention programmes that operate through diagnosis at health facilities. Similar considerations suggest that health education programmes will only be equitable if they are universal since they offer the largest benefit to those populations with the higher incidence of ill health, which are also poorer, have less education and less access to health services.

Universal coverage is most easily achieved through public sector interventions. In fact, there are several characteristics of school health and nutrition programmes that make a compelling case for public sector intervention. First, there may be treatment externalities where there are external benefits gained to others in addition to the benefit for the treated individual. This is clearly the case for communicable disease interventions, especially against worm infection. For example, a deworming programme in Kenya found a reduction in worm load among children who did not take part in the deworming programme but lived near schools that did. Secondly, some forms of intervention (such as vector control, health education campaigns, epidemiological surveillance, and interventions that have strong externalities) are almost pure public goods; that is, no one can be excluded from using the goods or service they deliver. Thus, the private sector is unlikely to compete to deliver these goods. Finally, there is typically little private demand for general preventive measures, such as information on the value of washing hands. None of this is an argument against a private sector role in service delivery, but it does suggest that private sector demand is likely to be greater in middle income populations and where demand has been created by public sector actions. As we shall see, this appears to be the case in practice.

International efforts to support school health and nutrition programmes

A major step forward in international coordination was achieved when a framework to "Focusing Resources on Effective School Health (FRESH)"[7] was developed jointly by UNESCO, WHO, UNICEF, Education International and the World Bank. This partnership effort was launched at the World Education Forum in Dakar in April 2000, which carried the clear message that good school health and nutrition is a key component of efforts to achieve EFA. Since then, UNESCO has adopted FRESH as one of its flagship programmes contributing to

EFA, and other agencies, including the World Food Programme, the Partnership for Child Development, and Save the Children (US), have joined the partnership.

The FRESH framework is based on good practice recognised by all the partners, and provides a consensus approach for the effective implementation of health and nutrition services within school health and nutrition programmes. The framework calls for four core components to be made available, together, in all schools:

- *Policy*: health and nutrition related school policies that provide a non-discriminatory, safe and secure environment.
- *School environment*: access to safe water, and provision of separate sanitation facilities for girls and boys.
- *Education*: skills-based education that addresses health, nutrition and hygiene issues, and promotes positive behaviours.
- *Services*: simple, safe and familiar health and nutrition services that can be delivered cost-effectively in schools (such as deworming, micronutrient supplements, and snacks that avoid hunger), and increased access to youth-friendly clinics.

Adoption of this framework does not imply that these core components and strategies are the only important elements, but that implementing all of these in all schools would provide a sound initial basis for any pro-poor school health and nutrition programme. Furthermore, these components can be implemented effectively only if supported by strategic partnerships between: 1) the health and education sectors, especially teachers and health workers; 2) schools and the community; and 3) pupils and other stakeholders.

The common focus has encouraged concerted action by the participating agencies. It has also provided a common platform upon which to build agency-specific programmes, such as the "health promoting schools" initiative of WHO and the "child-friendly" schools of UNICEF. But perhaps the most important consequence of FRESH has been to offer a common "point of entry" for new efforts to improve health in schools. The following three examples of new international initiatives show how specific school health and nutrition interventions can be inserted into one or all of the four core components (policy, environment, education and services) of the FRESH framework.

- The multi-agency effort to *"Accelerate the Education Sector Response to HIV&AIDS in Africa"*, promotes the FRESH framework specifically, and encourages education systems to: 1) adopt *policies* that avoid HIV&AIDS discrimination and stigmatisation; 2) provide life-skills *education* programmes in schools to promote positive sexual and social behaviours; and 3) improve access to youth-friendly health *services*. More than 37 countries, and a similar number of agencies and NGOs, have collaborated in this effort since November 2002.

- The *"Food for Education"* initiative of the World Food Programme has gone beyond the provision of food aid to develop a programmatic link between nutrition and education, by promoting: 1) *policies* that make food aid conditional upon girls' participation in education; 2) nutrition *education* that improves the quality of students' diets; and 3) nutrition *services* that include deworming and the alleviation of short-term hunger. More than 30 countries have begun to implement these reforms since 2002.
- The *"Partners for Parasite Control (PPC)"*, led by WHO, promotes public and private efforts to include deworming in school health *services,* following a resolution of the 54th World Health Assembly to provide, by 2010, regular deworming treatment to 75 per cent of school-age children at risk (an estimated target population of 398 million). Nineteen of 41 target countries in Africa have begun school-based deworming programmes since 2001.

This consensus approach has increased significantly the number of countries implementing school health reforms, and the simplicity of the approach has helped ensure that these programmes go to scale. As a result of concerted action by governments and participating agencies, national programmes based on the FRESH framework have been adopted by over 24 countries in sub-Saharan Africa, targeting a population of 45 million school-age children.

Programmatic approaches in practice

The FRESH framework provides strategic guidance for the design of programmes to improve the education, health and nutrition of school-age children. But there is considerable variation in the practical design of actual programmes, reflecting differences in local needs and capacity. In a majority of cases, school health and nutrition programmes are delivered and funded by the public education sector, with a formal role for the health sector in design and supervision. In some countries, it was considered too difficult to immediately incorporate school health within the existing education system, and a more-or-less separate and time-bound school health and nutrition programme was established to initiate a process of progressively handing over responsibility to the education sector.

While this public sector "mainstream" model has proven the most popular, it is not the only successful approach. In some cases, the public sector has identified appropriate options and developed operational manuals, but then used a social fund to provide direct support to communities and schools to select and implement the most relevant actions locally, often with the assistance of NGOs.

In some middle income countries the move towards a demand-led approach has gone even further, with NGOs providing a private sector service dependent upon the contributions of parents or guardians.

Table 7.1 gives examples from several low and middle income countries that have been selected to illustrate this diversity, and to show how the four core components of FRESH are being supported by these different approaches.

Table 7.1. How FRESH is used in low and middle income countries.

Approach	Social fund: Public sector support for community intervention.	Private sector: Community payment for NGO implemented intervention.
Country examples	Tajikistan	Indonesia
Policy	The Ministry of Labour and Social Protection, with the Ministries of Education and of Health, have developed a Memorandum of Understanding that sets out health policies for the education sector. The programme channels resources through PTAs, which identify and assist needy children. A training programme, delivered by NGOs, prepares PTA members to develop proposals of up to US$5,000 for their school, to support activities selected from a menu of items.	The NGO *Yayasan Kusuma Buana* has a formal agreement with the education department in Jakarta and three other major cities to train teachers, perform diagnostic tests, and provide medicines and materials. The NGO offers Pap smear tests and referral services to teachers. Unit costs are low because parasite diagnosis involves mass screening in a central laboratory (approximately 2,500 diagnoses per day), and medicines are obtained at preferential rates from two commercial partners.
Environment	Provision of sanitation facilities, potable water, sports facilities.	Not included in programme.
Health education	Training of teachers in health promotion.	Nutrition and hygiene education as part of the curriculum.
Health services	Training of teachers to provide first aid, micronutrients and deworming; provision of food preparation facilities.	Stool examination by the laboratory, and deworming by teachers as necessary twice a year; iron folate provided by teachers twice a year (for 3 months).
Outcomes	The programme targets the 100,000 neediest children in all 200 schools in the 6 poorest districts of Tajikistan, at an approximate per capita cost of US$1.00 pa.	The programme has been in existence for 17 years and currently reaches 627 schools and 161,000 students, at a cost to parents of US$0.10 pa.

Table 7.1. *continued.* How FRESH is used in low and middle income countries.

	Public sector: Public sector supported and implemented.	Programme approach: Parastatal support for public sector intervention.
Approach		
Country examples	Guinea, Ghana and Tanzania	Madagascar
Policy	In all three countries, the Ministry of Education (or in Ghana, its executive body, the Ghana Education Service) implements the programme under the guidance of the Ministry of Health, based on a formal policy agreement. In Tanzania the Ministries of Community Development and of Local Government are also parties to the agreement. The existing in-service teacher training and supply line infrastructures are used to prepare teachers and supply the necessary materials.	The community nutrition programme (SEECALINE II) provides training and support to the Ministry of Education, based on a formally agreed health policy for the education sector. In all schools in the 43 poorest districts (44% of all districts), the programme prepares teachers, and provides materials. In addition, the programme also provides PTAs with access to a social fund to support construction of facilities. Each PTA can request up to US$500 with a 20% community contribution based on a parental contribution of US$0.16 pa.
Environment	Separate sanitation facilities for girls and boys in all new schools; access to potable water in all schools.	Access to potable water, hand-washing facilities, in all schools; where requested by PTAs, construction of latrines, wells, fences and sports facilities.
Health education	Health, hygiene and nutrition education as part of the formal curriculum.	A formal health education curriculum, supported by community IEC.
Health services	Deworming (for both schistosomiasis and intestinal worms) provided by teachers twice a year; in Guinea this is followed by iron folate supplementation.	Twice yearly deworming and iron folate (for 3 months) delivered by teachers; tests kits to confirm iodisation of local sources of salt: where requested by PTAs, provision of food preparation facilities.
Outcomes	In three years, the Guinea programme has reached 600 schools and 350,000 students, the Ghana programme 577 schools and 83,000 students (at a cost of US$0.54 per child treated), and the Tanzania programme 353 schools and 113,000 students (at a cost of US$0.89 per child treated).	In three years, the programme has trained 14,000 teachers and in 4,585 schools, and reached 430,000 students at an estimated cost of US$0.78 to US$1.08 per capita pa.

Analysis of reports of school health and nutrition programmes from 40 low and middle income countries indicates that some 85 per cent have adopted the "mainstream" public sector model. Annual external support for these actions is currently approaching US$90 million, targeting some 100 million schoolchildren. The remaining countries have chosen programme- or social fund-based approaches, with a minority implementing the private sector option.

The private sector approach has proven sustainable over nearly two decades in urban Indonesia, but may require a technical infrastructure and local market base that are inappropriate for predominantly rural low income countries. The approach is modelled on a programme initiated in Japan in 1948, which relied on private sector technicians, working independently at first but later formalised within the Japan Association of Parasite Control, who conducted stool examinations and then treated infected individuals for a per capita fee equivalent to approximately US$0.74 in 2004. With growing prosperity, Japan later implemented a sophisticated, comprehensive school health programme based on the 1958 School Health Act, but retained the parasite control element of the programme because of its remarkable cost-effectiveness. The prevalence of roundworm infection fell from a high of 73 per cent in 1949 to less than 0.01 per cent by 1985. At its peak, the private sector programme conducted some 12 million examinations annually, implying a turnover of nearly US$9 million at today's prices.

Lessons learned from programmatic experience

It is apparent that there are many ways to approach the delivery of school health and nutrition, but these diverse experiences do suggest some common features. In particular, there is consistency in the roles played by government and non-governmental agencies and other partners and stakeholders (Table 7.2).

In nearly every case, the Ministry of Education is the lead implementing agency, reflecting both the goal of school health and nutrition programmes in improving educational achievement and the fact that the education system provides the most complete existing infrastructure to reach school-age children. But the education sector must share this responsibility with the Ministry of Health, particularly since the latter has the ultimate responsibility for health of children, including schoolchildren. It is also apparent that programme success is dependent upon the effective participation of numerous other stakeholders, especially the beneficiaries and their parents or guardians. The children and their families are the clients of these programmes, and their support for programme implementation is critical to programme success.

Table 7.2. Roles of agencies, partners and stakeholders in school health and nutrition programmes.

Partner	Roles	Comments
Ministry of Education	• lead implementing agency • lead financial resource • education sector policy	• health and nutrition of schoolchildren is a priority for EFA • education policy defines school environment, curriculum, duties of teachers • the education system has a pervasive infrastructure for reaching teachers and school-age children
Ministry of Health	• lead technical agency • health sector policy	• health of school-age children has lower priority than clinical services, infant health • health policy defines role of teachers in service delivery, procurement of health materials
Other public sector agencies. (e.g. Welfare, Social Affairs, Local Govt.)	• support education and health systems • fund holders	• Ministries of Local Government are often fund holders for teachers and schools, and for clinics and health agents • Ministries of Welfare and Social Affairs provide mechanisms for the provision of social funds
Private sector (e.g. health service, pharmaceuticals, publications)	• specialist service delivery • material provision	• major roles in drug procurement and training materials production • specialist roles in health diagnostics
Civil society (e.g. NGOs, FBOs, PTAs)	• training and supervision • local resource provision	• at the local level, serve as gatekeepers and fund holders, and may target implementation • additional resource streams, particularly through INGOs
Teacher associations	• define teachers' roles	• school health programmes demand an expanded role for teachers
The community (children, teachers, parents)	• partners in implementation • define acceptability of curriculum and teachers' roles • supplement resources	• communities are gatekeepers for the content of health education (especially moral and sexual content) and for the role of non-health agents (especially teachers) in health service delivery. Pupils are active participants in all aspects of the process at the school level • communities supplement programme finance at the margins

Key issues in designing an effective school health and nutrition programme

The diverse experiences of school health and nutrition programming suggest some key elements which are common contributors to success in many programmes.

- **Focus on education outcomes:** Making an explicit link between school health and nutrition programmes and education sector priorities (especially EFA and gender equity), helps ensure the commitment of the sector to programme support and implementation.
- **Develop a formal, multi-sectoral policy:** Education sector actions in health require the explicit agreement of the health sector. This potential tension can be resolved by setting out sectoral responsibilities at the outset, while failure to enter into dialogue has led, in Africa and Central Asia, to some health sectors resisting teacher delivery of deworming drugs, despite WHO recommendations.
- **Initiate a process of wide dissemination and consultation:** There are multiple stakeholders, implementers, enablers and gatekeepers, and a process of consultation will establish ownership and identify obstacles before they constrain progress. The process should involve at least CBOs, NGOs, FBOs, the community, pupils and teacher associations. In one country in East Africa, lack of prior agreement on the content of sex education delayed implementation for more than 3 years.
- **Use the existing infrastructure as much as possible:** Building on existing curriculum opportunities and the network of teachers will accelerate implementation and reduce costs. Programmes which rely on the development of new delivery systems – mobile school health teams, a cadre of school nurses – are expensive and complicated to take to scale.
- **Build the programme around simple, safe and familiar health and nutrition interventions:** Success in rapidly reaching all schools is crucially dependent upon stakeholder acceptance, which is more likely if the interventions are already sanctioned by local and international agencies, and are already in common use by the community.
- **Provide primary support from public resources:** There are compelling arguments for public investment in school health and nutrition programmes: the contribution to economic growth, the high rate of return, the large externalities, and that the majority of interventions are public goods. On the other hand, there is evidence of market failure precluding private provision of programmes.
- **Be inclusive and innovative:** Although public resources are crucial for school health and nutrition programmes, contributions from outside the

public sector should not be excluded. NGOs have proven effective in supporting public sector programmes through training and supervision, particularly at the local level. While market failure has precluded the private sector from effectively implementing whole programmes, there are examples of successful contributions, particularly in dense urban populations and in middle income countries.

Building on such previous success can help bring the benefits of school health and nutrition programmes to the hundreds of millions of schoolchildren in need of them. Previous programmes demonstrate that there are many feasible ways for governments and agencies to act on the compelling case for school health and nutrition.

School health and nutrition programmes: a policy priority

The case for school health and nutrition programmes consists of several arguments, which have been developed in detail throughout this book. We now bring these arguments together under three key themes and conclude our case for school health and nutrition programmes.

School health and nutrition programmes improve equity in education

The reasons why school health and nutrition programmes improve equity in education cut across all aspects of these programmes and run through all chapters in this book. The arguments start with the pattern of disease prevalence around the world. The most common diseases of poor health and nutrition are highly concentrated among the poor. The argument continues with the impact such diseases have on education. The education of the poor and disadvantaged suffer the most from such diseases. Conversely, treating such diseases brings the greatest educational benefit for the poor. School health and nutrition programmes are unusual in this respect. Many other efforts to improve children's education result in better-off, more able children benefiting to the greatest extent. The argument for equitable outcomes concludes, and is put into action, through programmatic implementation. Interventions delivered through school-based programmes are able to reach the poor, rural communities that often have limited access to other health services. In this way, school health and nutrition programmes are able to target the poor more effectively, those who will reap the greatest educational benefits from improved health and nutrition.

School health and nutrition programmes can have a massive global impact

The global impact of school health and nutrition programmes is the product of the high prevalence of certain diseases and the substantial educational benefits of treating them. The major conditions of poor health and nutrition that affect children's education – iron deficiency anaemia, worm infections, malaria – are highly prevalent. Some diseases, such as worm infections, have the most ill effects in school-age children. Treating such diseases can have a surprisingly large impact on children's education, increasing the time they spend at school and their ability to learn while there. It also reinforces education efforts. Healthy children are more likely to benefit from improvements in education quality. Such educational benefits to good health when replicated across the vast numbers of children suffering from common illnesses could add up to a massive global impact of school health and nutrition programmes.

School health and nutrition programmes are a cost-effective "quick win"

All the major conditions of ill health and poor nutrition that affect education are preventable or treatable. In fact, many of them can be treated simply and cheaply. Intestinal worm infections can be controlled through a yearly or twice-yearly dose of deworming tablets; iron deficiency anaemia can be treated through weekly doses of iron supplementation. Such treatments are highly cost-effective as education interventions when implemented through the school system, significantly reducing delivery costs, with significant savings made possible by using interventions through the school system. Compared to many other education interventions, school health and nutrition programmes deliver similar education benefits for a much lower cost. In the complex set of conditions required for a child to learn well, improved health and nutrition is one of the simplest and cheapest to achieve.

These three arguments combine to make a compelling case for school health and nutrition programmes. The first two arguments – the potential for a massive global impact and the rare opportunity to improve equity in educational opportunities through simple interventions – both argue that school health and nutrition programmes are an important education policy option that should receive our attention. The third argument – the cost-effectiveness of school health and nutrition interventions – makes these programmes an urgent policy priority. They are an easy win in the attempts to deliver a quality education to all children around the world and should be implemented wherever they are needed. School health and nutrition programmes are not the solution to global educational challenges, but no solution can be complete without them. They are not merely an additional social benefit to attending school; they are an integral part of efforts to get children into school, and to help them learn while there. School health and nutrition programmes are essential for achieving Education for All.

References

Chapter 1

1. UNESCO, *The Dakar Framework for Action: Education for All – Meeting our collective commitments*. 2000, UNESCO: World Education Forum, Dakar.
2. United Nations, *General Assembly Resolution. Road Map towards the implementation of the United Nations Millennium declaration. Fifty-sixth session. Item 40 of the provisional agenda. Follow-up of the outcome of the Millennium summit.*, in *Report of the Secretary General*. 2001, United Nations: New York.
3. UN Millennium Project. *Quick wins*. 2000, Available from: http://www.unmillenniumproject.org/documents/4-MP-QuickWins-E.pdf.
4. Parker, S., S. Greer, and B. Zuckerman, *Double Jeopardy – The impact of poverty on early child-development*. Pediatric Clinics of North America, 1988. 35(6): p. 1227-1240.
5. Sen, A., *Development as freedom*. 1999, Oxford: Oxford University Press.
6. Kremer, M., *Randomised evaluations of educational programmes in developing countries: Some lessons*. American Economic Review, 2003. 93(2): p. 102-106.
7. Muralidharan, K., and V. Sundararaman, *Teacher incentives in developing countries: Experimental evidence from India*. 2006.
8. Youngson, R.M., *Collins dictionary of medicine*. 1992, Glasgow: Harper Collins.
9. Marshall, S.J., *Developing countries face double burden of disease*. Bulletin of the World Health Organisation, 2004. 82(7): p. 556-556.

Chapter 2

1. US Census Bureau, *Population Division, International Programmes Centre*. 2002.
2. Shann, F., *Etiology of severe pneumonia in children in developing countries*. Pediatric Infectious Disease Journal, 1986. 5(2): p. 247-252.
3. CDC, *Pneumonia among children in developing countries*. 2003.
4. Parashar, U.D., J.S. Bresee, and R.I. Glass, *The global burden of diarrhoeal disease in children*. Bulletin of the World Health Organisation, 2003. 81(4): p. 236-236.

5. WHO, *World Health Report: Changing history*. 2004, World Health Organisation: Geneva.

6. UNICEF, *State of the world's children — Childhood under threat*. 2005, UNICEF: New York.

7. WHO, *Antimalarial drug combination therapy: Report of a WHO technical consultation, Geneva, 4-5 April 2001*. 2001, WHO: Geneva.

8. Perry, R.T., and N.A. Halsey, *The clinical significance of measles: A review*. Journal of Infectious Diseases, 2004. 189: p. S4-S16.

9. Wanyama, C., *Africa's largest measles vaccination campaign could reduce childhood mortality by 20%*. Bulletin of the World Health Organisation, 2002. 80(12): p. 989-989.

10. UNAIDS, *Paediatric HIV infection and AIDS. UNAIDS Point of View*. 2002, UNAIDS: Geneva.

11. UNAIDS, *Report on the global HIV&AIDS epidemic: The Barcelona Report*. 2002, UNAIDS: Geneva.

12. de Onis, M., M. Blossner, E. Borghi, E.A. Frongillo, and R. Morris, *Estimates of global prevalence of childhood underweight in 1990 and 2015*. Jama-Journal of the American Medical Association, 2004. 291(21): p. 2600-2606.

13. UNICEF, *State of the world's children*. 2000, UNICEF: New York.

14. UNICEF, *State of the world's children — Nutrition*. 1998, UNICEF: New York.

15. Bundy, D.A.P., and H.L. Guyatt, *Schools for health: Focus on health, education and the school-age child*. Parasitology Today, 1996. 12(8): p. 1-16.

16. Drake, L.J., C. Maier, M.C.H. Jukes, A. Patrikios, D.A.P. Bundy, A. Gardner, and C. Dolan, *School-age children: Their health and nutrition*. Sub-Committee on Nutrition News, 2002. 25.

17. Drake, L.J., M.C.H. Jukes, R.J. Sternberg, and D.A.P. Bundy, *Geohelminthiasis (Ascariasis, Trichuriasis and hookworm): Cognitive and developmental impact*. Seminars in Pediatric Infectious Disease, 2000. 11(4): p. 1-9.

18. Partnership for Child Development, *Better health, nutrition and education for the school-aged child*. Transactions of the Royal Society of Tropical Medicine and Hygiene, 1997. 91: p. 1-2.

19. Chan, M.S., *The global burden of intestinal nematode infections: 50 years on*. Parasitology Today, 1997. 13(11): p. 438-443.

20. Bundy, D.A.P., *This wormy world — Then and now*. Parasitology Today, 1997. 13(11): p. 407-408.

21. Bundy, D.A.P., and G.F. Medley, *Immuno-epidemiology of human Geohelminthiasis — Ecological and immunological determinants of worm burden*. Parasitology, 1992. 104: p. S105-S119.

22. World Bank, *World Development Report: Investing in health*. 1993, Oxford: Oxford University Press.

23. Drake, L.J., and D.A.P. Bundy, *Multiple helminth infections in children: Impact and control*. Parisitology, 2001. 122: p. 573-581.

24. Bundy, D.A.P., A. Hall, G.F. Medley, and L. Savioli, *Evaluating measures to control intestinal parasitic infections*. World Health Statistics Quarterly, 1992. 45: p. 168-179.

25. Bundy, D.A.P., S. Lwin, J.S. Osika, J. McLaughlin, and C.O. Pannenborg, *What should schools do about malaria?* Parasitology Today, 2000. 16(5): p. 181-182.

26.   Clarke, S.E., S. Brooker, J.K. Njagi, E. Njau, B. Estambale, E. Muchiri, and P. Magnussein, *Malaria morbidity amongst schoolchildren living in two areas of contrasting transmission in Western Kenya*. American Journal of Tropical Medicine and Hygiene, in press.

27.   Murray, C., and A. Lopez, eds. *The global burden of disease: Global burden of disease and injury series. Volume I*. 1996, Harvard University Press: Boston: Harvard School of Public Health.

28.   Brooker, S., H. Guyatt, J. Omumbo, R. Shretta, L.J. Drake, and J. Ouma, *Situation analysis of malaria in school-aged children in Kenya — What can be done?* Parasitology Today, 2000. 16(5): p. 183-186.

29.   World Bank, *Education and HIV&AIDS: A Window of Hope*. 2002, The World Bank: Washington, DC.

30.   UNICEF/UNAIDS, *Children orphaned by AIDS: front-line responses from Eastern and Southern Africa*. 1999, UNICEF: New York.

31.   Gachuhi, D., *The impact of HIV&AIDS on education systems in the Eastern and Southern Africa region and the response of education systems to HIV&AIDS: Life skills programmes*. 1999, UNICEF: New York.

32.   Hunter, S., and J. Williamson, *Children on the brink: Strategies to support a generation isolated by HIV&AIDS*. 2002, UNAIDS/USAID: New York.

33.   Partnership for Child Development, *The health and nutritional status of schoolchildren in Africa: Evidence from school-based health programmes in Ghana and Tanzania*. Transactions of the Royal Society of Tropical Medicine and Hygiene, 1998. 93: p. 254-261.

34.   UNAIDS, *Epidemiological fact sheets*. 2000, UNAIDS: Geneva.

35.   Draper, A., *Child development and iron deficiency. Early action is critical for healthy mental, physical and social development*. 1997, INACG.

36.   Hall, A., L.J. Drake, and D.A.P. Bundy, *Public health measures to control helminth infections that contribute to iron deficiency anaemia*, in *Nutritional anaemias*. 2000, CRS Press LLC. p. 215-239.

37.   Brock, C., and N. Cammish, *Factors affecting female participation in seven countries*. 1997, DFID: London.

38.   Del Rosso, J.M., and T. Marek, *Class action: Improving school performance in the developing world through better health and nutrition*. 1996, The World Bank: Washington, DC.

39.   Partnership for Child Development, *Anaemia in schoolchildren in eight countries in Africa and Asia*. Public Health Nutrition, 2001. 4(3): p. 749-756.

40.   Lwenje, S.M., J.O. Okonkwo, V.S.B. Mtetwa, A.G. Gamedze, J.A. Mavundla, and M.M. Sihlongonyane, *Determination of urinary iodine in schoolchildren of the Hhohho region in Swaziland*. International Journal of Environmental Health Research, 1999. 9: p. 207-211.

41.   Kalk, W.J., J. Paiker, M.G. van Arb, and W. Pick, *Dietary iodine deficiency in South Africa*. South African Medical Journal, 1998. 88(3): p. 357-358.

42.   El-Sayed, N.A., A.A.R. Mahfouz, L. Nofal, H.M. Ismail, A. Gad, and H.A. Zeid, *Iodine deficiency disorders among schoolchildren in upper Egypt: An epidemiologic study*. Journal of Tropical Pediatrics, 1998. 44: p. 270-274.

43.   Del Rosso, J.M., *School feeding programmes: Improving effectiveness and increasing benefit to education*. 1999, Partnership for Child Development: London.

44.   WHO. *Combating vitamin A deficiency.* 2003 [cited 2007 31st March]; Available
        from: http://www.who.int/nutrition/vad.htm.
45.   Martorell, R., *Obesity in the developing world*, in *The Nutrition Transition: Diet-
        related diseases in the modern world*, B. Caballero and B.M. Popkin, Editors.
        2002.

Chapter 3

1.   UNESCO, *EFA Global Monitoring Report 2007: Strong foundations. Early
        childhood care and education.* 2007, UNESCO: Paris.
2.   UNESCO, *EFA Global Monitoring Report 2005: The quality imperative.* 2005,
        UNESCO: Paris.
3.   DFID, *The challenge of universal primary education: Strategies for achieving the
        international development targets.* 2001, DFID: London.
4.   Durkin, M., *The epidemiology of developmental disabilities in low-income
        countries.* Mental Retardation and Developmental Disabilities Research
        Reviews, 2002. 8(3): p. 206-211.
5.   Christianson, A.L., M.E. Zwane, R. Manga, E. Rosen, A. Venter, and J.G.R.
        Kromberg, *Epilepsy in rural South African children — Prevalence, associated
        disability and management.* South African Medical Journal, 2000. 90(3): p.
        262-266.
6.   Cao, X.Y., X.M. Jiang, Z.H. Dou, M.A. Rakeman, M.L. Zhang, K. Odonnell, T.
        Ma, K. Amette, N. Delong, and G.R. Delong, *Timing of vulnerability of the
        brain to iodine deficiency in endemic cretinism.* New England Journal of
        Medicine, 1994. 331(26): p. 1739-1744.
7.   Hetzel, B.S., *Iodine and neuropsychological development.* Journal of Nutrition,
        2000. 130(2): p. 493S-495S.
8.   Buccimazza, S.S., C.D. Molteno, T.T. Dunne, and D.L. Viljoen, *Prevalence of
        neural-tube defects in Cape Town, South Africa.* Teratology, 1994. 50(3): p.
        194-199.
9.   Wald, N., *Prevention of neural-tube defects — Results of the Medical Research
        Council vitamin study.* Lancet, 1991. 338(8760): p. 131-137.
10.   Mendez, M.A., and L.S. Adair, *Severity and timing of stunting in the first two
        years of life affect performance on cognitive tests in late childhood.* Journal of
        Nutrition, 1999. 129(8): p. 1555-1562.
11.   Cutts, F.T., and E. Vynnycky, *Modelling the incidence of congenital rubella
        syndrome in developing countries.* International Journal of Epidemiology,
        1999. 28(6): p. 1176-1184.
12.   Walker, D.G., and G.J.A. Walker, *Forgotten but not gone: The continuing
        scourge of congenital syphilis.* Lancet Infectious Diseases, 2002. 2(7): p. 432-
        436.
13.   Enders, M., and H.J. Hagedorn, *Syphilis in pregnancy.* Zeitschrift Fur
        Geburtshilfe Und Neonatologie, 2002. 206(4): p. 131-137.
14.   Watson-Jones, D., B. Gumodoka, H. Weiss, J. Changalucha, J. Todd, K. Mugeye,
        A. Buve, Z. Kanga, L. Ndeki, M. Rusizoka, D. Ross, J. Marealle, R. Balira, D.
        Mabey, and R. Hayes, *Syphilis in pregnancy in Tanzania II. The effectiveness
        of antenatal syphilis screening and single-dose benzathine penicillin
        treatment for the prevention of adverse pregnancy outcomes.* Journal of
        Infectious Diseases, 2002. 186(7): p. 948-957.

15. Murphy, S.C., and J.G. Breman, *Gaps in the childhood malaria burden in Africa: Cerebral malaria, neurological sequelae, anaemia, respiratory distress, hypoglycaemia, and complications of pregnancy.* American Journal of Tropical Medicine and Hygiene, 2001. 64(1-2): p. 57-67.

16. Brewster, D.R., D. Kwiatkowski, and N.J. White, *Neurological sequelae of cerebral malaria in children.* Lancet, 1990. 336(8722): p. 1039-1043.

17. Holding, P.A., H.G. Taylor, S.D. Kazungu, T. Mkala, J. Gona, B. Mwamuye, L. Mbonani, and J. Stevenson, *Assessing cognitive outcomes in a rural African population: Development of a neuropsychological battery,* in press.

18. Jukes, M.C.H., M. Pinder, E.L. Grigorenko, H.B. Smith, G. Walraven, E.M. Bariau, R.J. Sternberg, L.J. Drake, P. Milligan, Y.B. Cheung, B.M. Greenwood, and D.A.P. Bundy, *Long-term impact of malaria chemoprophylaxis on cognitive abilities and educational attainment: Follow-up of a controlled trial.* PLoS Clinical Trials, 2006. 1(4): p. e19.

19. Goetghebuer, T., T.E. West, V. Wermenbol, A.L. Cadbury, P. Milligan, N. Lloyd-Evans, R.A. Adegbola, E.K. Mulholland, B.M. Greenwood, and M.W. Weber, *Outcome of meningitis caused by Streptococcus pneumoniae and Haemophilus influenzae type b in children in The Gambia.* Tropical Medicine and International Health, 2000. 5(3): p. 207-213.

20. Glewwe, P., and H.G. Jacoby, *An economic-analysis of delayed primary school enrolment in a low income country − The role of early childhood nutrition.* Review of Economics and Statistics, 1995. 77(1): p. 156-169.

21. Jamison, D.T., *Child malnutrition and school performance in China.* Journal of Development Economics, 1986. 20(2): p. 299-309.

22. Moock, P.R., and J. Leslie, *Childhood malnutrition and schooling in the Terai region of Nepal.* Journal of Development Economics, 1986. 20(1): p. 33-52.

23. Partnership for Child Development, *Short stature and the age of enrolment in primary school: Studies in two African countries.* Social Science and Medicine, 1999. 48: p. 675-682.

24. Alderman, H., J.R. Behrman, V. Lavy, and R. Menon, *Child health and school enrolment − A longitudinal analysis.* Journal of Human Resources, 2001. 36(1): p. 185-205.

25. Jukes, M.C.H., *Associations between nutritional status and practical activities of school-age children in Tanzania,* in press.

26. Cueto, S., *Heights and weights as predictors or achievement, grade repetition and drop-out in two samples in rural Peru.* in *Schoolchildren: Health and nutrition.* 2004, University of California, Los Angeles.

27. Montresor, A., M. Ramsan, H.M. Chwaya, H. Ameir, A. Foum, M. Albonico, T.W. Gyorkos, and L. Savioli, *School enrolment in Zanzibar linked to children's age and helminth infections.* Tropical Medicine and International Health, 2001. 6(3): p. 227-231.

28. Beasley, N.M.R., A. Hall, A.M. Tomkins, C. Donnelly, P. Ntimbwa, J. Kivuga, C.M. Kihamia, W. Lorri, and D.A.P. Bundy, *The health of enrolled and non-enrolled children of school-age in Tanga, Tanzania.* Acta Tropica, 2000. 76(3): p. 223-229.

29. Leighton, C., and R. Foster, *Economic impacts of malaria in Kenya and Nigeria,* in *HFS Applied Research Paper.* 1993, Bethesda.

30. Trape, J.F., E. Lefebvrezante, F. Legros, P. Druilhe, C. Rogier, H. Bouganali, and G. Salem, *Malaria morbidity among children exposed to low seasonal*

transmission in Dakar, Senegal and its implications for malaria control in tropical Africa. American Journal of Tropical Medicine and Hygiene, 1993. 48(6): p. 748-756.

31.   Brooker, S., H. Guyatt, J. Omumbo, R. Shretta, L.J. Drake, and J. Ouma, *Situation analysis of malaria in school-aged children in Kenya — What can be done?* Parasitology Today, 2000. 16(5): p. 183-186.

32.   Colbourne, M.J., *The effect of malaria suppression in a group of Accra schoolchildren.* Transactions of the Royal Society of Tropical Medicine and Hygiene, 1955. 49: p. 356-369.

33.   Fernando, D., D. De Silva, R. Carter, K.N. Mendis, and R. Wickremasinghe, *A randomised, double-blind, placebo-controlled, clinical trial of the impact of malaria prevention on the educational attainment of schoolchildren.* American Journal of Tropical Medicine and Hygiene, 2006. 74(3): p. 386-393.

34.   Shiff, C., W. Checkley, P. Winch, Z. Premji, J. Minjas, and P. Lubega, *Changes in weight gain and anaemia attributable to malaria in Tanzanian children living under holoendemic conditions.* Transactions of the Royal Society of Tropical Medicine and Hygiene, 1996. 90(3): p. 262-265.

35.   Hutchinson, S.E., C.A. Powell, S.P. Walker, S.M. Chang, and S.M. Grantham-McGregor, *Nutrition, anaemia, geohelminth infection and school achievement in rural Jamaican primary schoolchildren.* European Journal of Clinical Nutrition, 1997. 51(11): p. 729-735.

36.   Nokes, C., and D.A.P. Bundy, *Compliance and absenteeism in schoolchildren: implications for helminth control.* Transactions of the Royal Society of Tropical Medicine and Hygiene, 1993. 87: p. 148-152.

37.   de Clercq, D., M. Sacko, J. Behnke, F. Gilbert, and J. Vercruysse, *The relationship between Schistosoma haematobium infection and school performance and attendance in Bamako, Mali.* Annals of Tropical Medicine and Parasitology, 1998. 92(8): p. 851-858.

38.   Simeon, D.T., S.M. Grantham-McGregor, J.E. Callender, and M.S. Wong, *Treatment of Trichuris trichiura infections improves growth, spelling scores and school attendance in some children.* Journal of Nutrition, 1995. 125(7): p. 1875-1883.

39.   Miguel, E., and M. Kremer, *Worms: Identifying impacts on education and health in the presence of treatment externalities.* Econometrica, 2004. 72(1): p. 159-217.

40.   Bobonis, G., E. Miguel, and C. Sharma, *Iron deficiency anaemia and school performance.* submitted.

41.   Vermeersch, C., and M. Kremer, *School meals, educational achievement, and school competition: Evidence from a randomised evaluation,* in *The World Bank Policy Research Working Paper No. 3523.* 2004, The World Bank: Washington, DC.

42.   Yoshizawa, K., and A.A. Mon, *Nutritional status of children by school attendance in Myanmar.* Faseb Journal, 2002. 16(4): p. A278-A278.

43.   Powell, C.A., S.P. Walker, S.M. Chang, and S.M. Grantham-McGregor, *Nutrition and education: A randomised trial of the effects of breakfast in rural primary schoolchildren.* American Journal of Clinical Nutrition, 1998. 68: p. 873-879.

44.   van Stuijvenberg, M.E., J.D. Kvalsvig, M. Faber, M. Kruger, D.G. Kenoyer, and A.J.S. Benade, *Effect of iron-, iodine-, and beta-carotene-fortified biscuits on*

the micronutrient status of primary schoolchildren: A randomised controlled trial. American Journal of Clinical Nutrition, 1999. 69(3): p. 497-503.

45.   Evans, D.K., and E. Miguel, *Orphans and schooling in Africa: A longitudinal analysis.* Demography, 2007. 44(1): p. 35-57.

46.   Harris, A.M., and J.G. Schubert, *Defining 'quality' in the midst of HIV&AIDS: Ripple effects in the classroom. IEQ project.* in *44th Annual Meeting of the Comparative Education Society.* 2001, Washington, DC.

47.   Ainsworth, M., K. Beegle, and G. Koda, *The impact of adult mortality on primary school enrolment in North-Western Tanzania.* 2001, UNAIDS: Geneva.

48.   Nyamukapa, C., and S. Gregson, *Extended family's and women's roles in safeguarding orphans' education in AIDS-afflicted rural Zimbabwe.* Social Science and Medicine, 2005. 60(10): p. 2155-2167.

49.   Liddell, C., and G. Rae, *Predicting early grade retention: A longitudinal investigation of primary school progress in a sample of rural South African children.* British Journal of Educational Psychology, 2001. 71: p. 413-428

Chapter 4

1.   Dauncey, M.J., and R.J. Bicknell, *Nutrition and neurodevelopment: Mechanisms of developmental dysfunction and disease in later life.* Nutrition Research Reviews, 1999. 12(2): p. 231-253.

2.   Boivin, M.J., *Effects of early cerebral malaria on cognitive ability in Senegalese children.* Journal of Developmental and Behavioural Pediatrics, 2002. 23(5): p. 353-364.

3.   Watkins, W.E., and E. Pollitt, *Stupidity or worms: Do intestinal worms impair mental performance?* Psychological Bulletin, 1997. 121: p. 171-191.

4.   Lozoff, B., G.M. Brittenham, A.W. Wolf, D.K. McClish, P.M. Kuhnert, E. Jimenez, R. Jimenez, L.A. Mora, I. Gomez, and D. Krauskoph, *Iron deficiency anaemia and iron therapy effects on infant developmental test performance [published erratum appears in Pediatrics 1988 May;81(5):683].* Pediatrics, 1987. 79(6): p. 981-995.

5.   Kandel, E.R., J.H. Schwartz, and T.M. Jessell, *Principles of neural science.* Fourth Edition. 2000, London: McGraw-Hill.

6.   Grantham-McGregor, S.M., W. Schofield, and D. Haggard, *Maternal–child interaction in survivors of severe malnutrition who received psychosocial stimulation.* European Journal of Clinical Nutrition, 1989. 43(1): p. 45-52.

7.   Hippocrates, *Hippocrates. Volume. 2.* 1923, London and New York: William Heinemann and Harvard University Press.

8.   Peeling, A.N., and J.L. Smart, *Review of literature showing that undernutrition affects the growth rate of all processes in the brain to the same extent [see comments].* Metabolic Brain Disease, 1994. 9(1): p. 33-42.

9.   Smart, J.L., *Vulnerability of developing brain to undernutrition.* Upsala Journal of Medical Sciences, 1990: p. 21-41.

10.   Simeon, D., and S.M. Grantham-McGregor, *Nutritional deficiencies and children's behaviour and mental development.* Nutrition Research Reviews, 1990. 3: p. 1-24.

11.   Lasky, R.E., R.E. Klein, C. Yarbrough, P.L. Engle, A. Lechtig, and R. Martorell, *The relationship between physical growth and infant behavioural*

development in rural Guatemala. Child Development, 1981. 52(1): p. 219-226.

12.   Whaley, S.E., M. Sigman, M.P. Espinosa, and C.G. Neumann, *Infant predictors of cognitive development in an undernourished Kenyan population.* Journal of Developmental and Behavioural Pediatrics, 1998. 19(3): p. 169-177.

13.   Grantham-McGregor, S.M., *A review of studies of the effect of severe malnutrition on mental development.* Journal of Nutrition, 1995. 125(8 Suppl): p. 2233s-2238s.

14.   Grantham-McGregor, S.M., M. Stewart, and P. Desai, *A new look at the assessment of mental development in young children recovering from severe malnutrition.* Developmental Medicine & Child Neurology, 1978. 20(6): p. 773-778.

15.   Grantham-McGregor, S.M., C. Powell, and P. Fletcher, *Stunting, severe malnutrition and mental development in young children.* European Journal of Clinical Nutrition, 1989. 43(6): p. 403-409.

16.   Joos, S.K., E. Pollitt, W.H. Mueller, and D.L. Albright, *The bacon chow study: Maternal nutritional supplementation and infant behavioural development.* Child Development, 1983. 54(3): p. 669-676.

17.   Freeman, H.E., R.E. Klein, J.W. Townsend, and A. Lechtig, *Nutrition and cognitive development among rural Guatemalan children.* American Journal of Public Health, 1980. 70(12): p. 1277-1285.

18.   Chavez, A., and C. Martinez, *School performance of supplemented and unsupplemented children from a poor rural area.* Progress in Clinical and Biological Research, 1981. 77: p. 393-402.

19.   Waber, D.P., L. Vuori-Christiansen, N. Ortiz, J.R. Clement, N.E. Christiansen, J.O. Mora, R.B. Reed, and M.G. Herrera, *Nutritional supplementation, maternal education, and cognitive development of infants at risk of malnutrition.* American Journal of Clinical Nutrition, 1981. 34(4): p. 807-813.

20.   Vermeersch, C., and M. Kremer, *School meals, educational achievement, and school competition: Evidence from a randomised evaluation,* in *World Bank Policy Research Working Paper No. 3523.* 2004, The World Bank: Washington, DC.

21.   Husaini, M.A., L. Karyadi, Y.K. Husaini, Sandjaja, D. Karyadi, and E. Pollitt, *Developmental effects of short-term supplementary feeding in nutritionally-at-risk Indonesian infants.* American Journal of Clinical Nutrition, 1991. 54(5): p. 799-804.

22.   McKay, H., L. Sinisterra, A. McKay, H. Gomez, and P. Lloreda, *Improving cognitive ability in chronically deprived children.* Science, 1978. 200 (4339): p. 270-278.

23.   Grantham-McGregor, S.M., C.A. Powell, S.P. Walker, and J.H. Himes, *Nutritional supplementation, psychosocial stimulation, and mental development of stunted children — The Jamaican study.* Lancet, 1991. 338(8758): p. 1-5.

24.   Grantham-McGregor, S.M., M.E. Stewart, and W.N. Schofield, *Effect of long-term psychosocial stimulation on mental development of severely malnourished children.* Lancet, 1980. 2(8198): p. 785-789.

25.   Grantham-McGregor, S.M., C.A. Powell, S. Walker, S.M. Chang, and P. Fletcher, *The long-term follow-up of severely malnourished children who participated in an intervention programme.* Child Development, 1994. 65(2): p. 428-439.

26.   Grantham-McGregor, S.M., S.P. Walker, S.M. Chang, and C.A. Powell, *Effects of early childhood supplementation with and without stimulation on later development in stunted Jamaican children.* American Journal of Clinical Nutrition, 1997. 66(2): p. 247-253.

27.   Walker, S.P., S.M. Grantham-McGregor, C.A. Powell, and S.M. Chang, *Effects of growth restriction in early childhood on growth, IQ, and cognition at age 11 to 12 years and the benefits of nutritional supplementation and psychosocial stimulation.* Journal of Pediatrics, 2000. 137(1): p. 36-41.

28.   Chang, S.M., S.P. Walker, S.M. Grantham-McGregor, and C.A. Powell, *Early childhood stunting and later behaviour and school achievement.* Journal of Child Psychology and Psychiatry and Allied Disciplines, 2002. 43(6): p. 775-783.

29.   Pollitt, E., K.S. Gorman, P.L. Engle, J.A. Rivera, and R. Martorell, *Nutrition in early life and the fulfilment of intellectual potential.* Journal of Nutrition, 1995. 125(4): p. S1111-S1118.

30.   Pollitt, E., W.E. Watkins, and M.A. Husaini, *Three-month nutritional supplementation in Indonesian infants and toddlers benefits memory function 8 years later.* American Journal of Clinical Nutrition, 1997. 66(6): p. 1357-1363.

31.   Watanabe, K., R. Flores, J. Fujiwara, and T.H.T. Lien, *Early childhood development interventions and cognitive development of young children in rural Vietnam.* Journal of Nutrition, 2005. 135(8): p. 1918-1925.

32.   Glewwe, P., and E.M. King, *The impact of early childhood nutritional status on cognitive development: Does the timing of malnutrition matter?* World Bank Economic Review, 2001. 15(1): p. 81-113.

33.   Mendez, M.A., and L.S. Adair, *Severity and timing of stunting in the first two years of life affect performance on cognitive tests in late childhood.* Journal of Nutrition, 1999. 129(8): p. 1555-1562.

34.   Wachs, T.D., M. Sigman, Z. Bishry, W. Moussa, N. Jerome, C. Neumann, N. Bwibo, and M.A. McDonald, *Caregiver child interaction patterns in two cultures in relation to nutritional intake.* International Journal of Behavioural Development, 1992. 15(1): p. 1-18.

35.   Cravioto, J., and R. Arrieta, *Stimulation and mental development of malnourished infants.* Lancet., 1979. 2(8148): p. 899.

36.   McDonald, M.A., M. Sigman, M.P. Espinosa, and C.G. Neumann, *Impact of a temporary food shortage on children and their mothers.* Child Development, 1994. 65(2): p. 404-415.

37.   Grantham-McGregor, S.M., *Small for gestational age, term babies, in the first six years of life.* European Journal of Clinical Nutrition, 1998. 52: p. S59-S64.

38.   Hack, M., *Effects of intrauterine growth retardation on mental performance and behaviour, outcomes during adolescence and adulthood.* European Journal of Clinical Nutrition, 1998. 52: p. S65-S71.

39.   Agarwal, K.N., D.K. Agarwal, and S.K. Upadhyay, *Impact of chronic undernutrition on higher mental functions in Indian boys aged 10-12 years.* Acta Paediatrica, 1995. 84(12): p. 1357-1361.

40.   UNICEF, *State of the world's children — Childhood under threat.* 2005, UNICEF: New York.

41. Anderson, J.W., B.M. Johnstone, and D.T. Remley, *Breast-feeding and cognitive development: A meta-analysis.* American Journal of Clinical Nutrition, 1999. 70(4): p. 525-535.

42. Angelsen, N.K., T. Vik, G. Jacobsen, and L.S. Bakketeig, *Breast-feeding and cognitive development at age 1 and 5 years.* Archives of Disease in Childhood, 2001. 85(3): p. 183-188.

43. Jain, A., J. Concato, and J.M. Leventhal, *How good is the evidence linking breast-feeding and intelligence?* Pediatrics, 2002. 109(6): p. 1044-1053.

44. Beard, J., *Iron deficiency alters brain development and functioning.* Journal of Nutrition, 2003. 133(5): p. 1468S-1472S.

45. Roncagliolo, M., M. Garrido, T. Walter, P. Peirano, and B. Lozoff, *Evidence of altered central nervous system development in infants with iron deficiency anaemia at 6 months: Delayed maturation of auditory brainstem responses.* American Journal of Clinical Nutrition, 1998. 68(3): p. 683-690.

46. Grantham-McGregor, S.M., and C. Ani, *A review of studies on the effect of iron deficiency on cognitive development in children.* Journal of Nutrition, 2001. 131(2): p. 649S-666S.

47. Walter, T., *Infancy — Mental and motor development.* American Journal of Clinical Nutrition, 1989. 50(3): p. 655-666.

48. Lozoff, B., G.M. Brittenham, F.E. Viteri, A.W. Wolf, and J.J. Urrutia, *The effects of short-term oral iron therapy on developmental deficits in iron deficient anaemic infants.* Journal of Pediatrics, 1982. 100(3): p. 351-357.

49. Idjradinata, P., and E. Pollitt, *Reversal of developmental delays in iron deficient anaemic infants treated with iron [see comments].* Lancet, 1993. 341(8836): p. 1-4.

50. Pollitt, E., C. Sacopollitt, R.L. Leibel, and F.E. Viteri, *Iron deficiency and behavioural development in infants and preschool children.* American Journal of Clinical Nutrition, 1986. 43(4): p. 555-565.

51. Soewondo, S., M. Husaini, and E. Pollitt, *Effects of iron deficiency on attention and learning processes in preschool children - Bandung, Indonesia.* American Journal of Clinical Nutrition, 1989. 50(3): p. 667-674.

52. Seshadri, S., and T. Gopaldas, *Impact of iron supplementation on cognitive functions in preschool and school-aged children: The Indian experience.* American Journal of Clinical Nutrition, 1989. 50(3 Suppl): p. 675-684.

53. Stoltzfus, R.J., J.D. Kvalsvig, H.M. Chwaya, A. Montresor, M. Albonico, J.M. Tielsch, L. Savioli, and E. Pollitt, *Iron improves language and motor development of African preschoolers.* Faseb Journal, 2001. 15(4): p. A254-A254.

54. Lozoff, B., E. Jimenez, J. Hagen, E. Mollen, and A.W. Wolf, *Poorer behavioural and developmental outcome more than 10 years after treatment for iron deficiency in infancy.* Pediatrics, 2000. 105(4): p. e51.

55. Lozoff, B., E. Jimenez, and A.W. Wolf, *Long-term developmental outcome of infants with iron deficiency.* New England Journal of Medicine, 1991. 325(10): p. 687-694.

56. de Andraca Oyarzun, I., B. Gonzalez Lopez, and M.I. Salas Aliaga, *[Characteristics of the family structure of schoolchildren with antecedents of severe and early malnutrition which nowadays present different intellectual levels].* Arch. Latinoam Nutrition, 1991. 41(2): p. 168-181.

57.   Palti, H., B. Pevsner, and B. Adler, *Does anaemia in infancy affect achievement on developmental and intelligence tests?* Human Biology, 1983. 55(1): p. 183-194.

58.   Palti, H., A. Meijer, and B. Adler, *Learning achievement and behaviour at school of anaemic and non-anaemic infants.* Early Human Development, 1985. 10(3-4): p. 217-223.

59.   Hurtado, E.K., A.H. Claussen, and K.G. Scott, *Early childhood anaemia and mild or moderate mental retardation.* American Journal of Clinical Nutrition, 1999. 69(1): p. 115-119.

60.   Delange, F., *The role of iodine in brain development.* Proceedings of the Nutrition Society, 2000. 59(1): p. 75-79.

61.   Boyages, S.C., and J.P. Halpern, *Endemic cretinism: Toward a unifying hypothesis.* Thyroid, 1993. 3(1): p. 59-69.

62.   Greene, L.S., *Iodine malnutrition, inbreeding, and developmental retardation.* American Journal of Physical Anthropology, 1984. 63(2): p. 166-166.

63.   Pharoah, P.O.D., and K.J. Connolly, *A controlled trial of iodinated oil for the prevention of endemic cretinism − A long-term follow-up.* International Journal of Epidemiology, 1987. 16(1): p. 68-73.

64.   Bleichrodt, N., and M.P. Born, *Iodine deficiency disorders: A meta-analysis.* International Journal of Psychology, 1996. 31(3-4): p. 5768-5768.

65.   Grant, E.C.G., J.M. Howard, S. Davies, H. Chasty, B. Hornsby, and J. Galbraith, *Zinc-deficiency in children with dyslexia − Concentrations of zinc and other minerals in sweat and hair.* British Medical Journal, 1988. 296(6622): p. 607-609.

66.   Grant, E.C.G., *Developmental dyslexia and zinc deficiency.* Lancet, 2004. 364(9430): p. 247-248.

67.   Hamadani, J.D., G.J. Fuchs, S.J.M. Osendarp, S.N. Huda, and S.M. Grantham-McGregor, *Zinc supplementation during pregnancy and effects on mental development and behaviour of infants: A follow-up study.* Lancet, 2002. 360(9329): p. 290-294.

68.   Hamadani, J.D., G.J. Fuchs, S.J.M. Osendarp, F. Khatun, S.N. Huda, and S.M. Grantham-McGregor, *Randomised controlled trial of the effect of zinc supplementation on the mental development of Bangladeshi infants.* American Journal of Clinical Nutrition, 2001. 74(3): p. 381-386.

69.   Gardner, J.M.M., C.A. Powell, H. Baker-Henningham, S.P. Walker, T.J. Cole, and S.M. Grantham-McGregor, *Zinc supplementation and psychosocial stimulation: Effects on the development of undernourished Jamaican children.* American Journal of Clinical Nutrition, 2005. 82(2): p. 399-405.

70.   Holding, P.A., J. Stevenson, N. Peshu, and K. Marsh, *Cognitive sequelae of severe malaria with impaired consciousness.* Transactions of the Royal Society of Tropical Medicine and Hygiene, 1999. 93(5): p. 529-534.

71.   Muntendam, A.H., S. Jaffar, N. Bleichrodt, and M.B. van Hensbroek, *Absence of neuropsychological sequelae following cerebral malaria in Gambian children.* Transactions of the Royal Society of Tropical Medicine and Hygiene, 1996. 90(4): p. 391-394.

72.   Holding, P.A., and R.W. Snow, *Impact of Plasmodium falciparum malaria on performance and learning: Review of the evidence.* American Journal of Tropical Medicine and Hygiene, 2001. 64(1-2): p. 68-75.

73. Jukes, M.C.H., M. Pinder, E.L. Grigorenko, H.B. Smith, G. Walraven, E.M. Bariau, R.J. Sternberg, L.J. Drake, P. Milligan, Y.B. Cheung, B.M. Greenwood, and D.A.P. Bundy, *Long-term impact of malaria chemoprophylaxis on cognitive abilities and educational attainment: Follow-up of a controlled trial.* PLoS Clinical Trials, 2006. 1(4): p. e19.

74. Sowunmi, A., *Psychosis after cerebral malaria in children.* Journal of the National Medical Association, 1993. 85(9): p. 695-696.

75. Sowunmi, A., J.U. Ohaeri, and C.O. Falade, *Falciparum malaria presenting as psychosis.* Tropical and Geographical Medicine, 1995. 47(5): p. 218-219.

76. Ansell, J., K.A. Hamilton, M. Pinder, G.E.L. Walraven, and S.W. Lindsay, *Short-range attractiveness of pregnant women to Anopheles Gambiae mosquitoes.* Transactions of the Royal Society of Tropical Medicine and Hygiene, 2002. 96(2): p. 113-116.

77. Brooker, S., N. Peshu, P.A. Warn, M. Mosobo, H.L. Guyatt, K. Marsh, and R.W. Snow, *The epidemiology of hookworm infection and its contribution to anaemia among preschool children on the Kenyan coast.* Transactions of the Royal Society of Tropical Medicine and Hygiene, 1999. 93(3): p. 240-246.

78. Stoltzfus, R.J., J.D. Kvalsvig, H.M. Chwaya, A. Montresor, M. Albonico, J.M. Tielsch, L. Savioli, and E. Pollitt, *Effects of iron supplementation and anthelmintic treatment on motor and language development of preschool children in Zanzibar: Double blind, placebo controlled study.* BMJ, 2001. 323(7326): p. 1389.

79. Jukes, M.C.H., C. Sharma, E. Miguel, and G. Bobonis, *The effect of iron supplementation on attention and cognitive development in Indian preschool children,* in prep.

80. Berkman, D.S., A.G. Lescano, R.H. Gilman, S. Lopez, and M.M. Black, *Effects of stunting, diarrhoeal disease, and parasitic infection during infancy on cognition in late childhood: A follow-up study.* Lancet, 2002. 359(9306): p. 564-571.

81. Berman, S., *Otitis media in developing countries.* Pediatrics, 1995. 96(1): p. 126-131.

82. Balle, V.H., M. Tos, D.H. Son, N.T. Son, L. Tri, T.K. Phoung, T.T.T. Mai, and V.M. Tien, *Prevalence of chronic otitis media in a randomly selected population from two communes in Southern Vietnam.* Acta Oto-Laryngologica, 2000: p. 51-53.

83. Rupa, V., A. Jacob, and A. Joseph, *Chronic suppurative otitis media: Prevalence and practices among rural South Indian children.* International Journal of Pediatric Otorhinolaryngology, 1999. 48(3): p. 217-221.

84. Casby, M.W., *Otitis media and language development: A meta-analysis.* American Journal of Speech-Language Pathology, 2001. 10(1): p. 65-80.

85. Roberts, J.E., M.R. Burchinal, S.A. Zeisel, E.C. Neebe, S.R. Hooper, J. Roush, D. Bryant, M. Mundy, and F.W. Henderson, *Otitis media, the care giving environment, and language and cognitive outcomes at 2 years.* Pediatrics, 1998. 102(2): p. 346-354.

86. Hodgson, A., T. Smith, S. Gagneux, I. Akumah, M. Adjuik, G. Pluschke, F. Binka, and B. Genton, *Infectious diseases — Survival and sequelae of meningococcal meningitis in Ghana.* International Journal of Epidemiology, 2001. 30(6): p. 1440-1446.

87.   Berg, S., B. Trollfors, S. Hugosson, E. Fernell, and E. Svensson, *Long-term follow-up of children with bacterial meningitis with emphasis on behavioural characteristics.* European Journal of Pediatrics, 2002. 161(6): p. 330-336.

88.   Koomen, I., D.E. Grobbee, A. Jennekens-Schinkel, J.J. Roord, and A.M. van Furth, *Parental perception of educational, behavioural and general health problems in school-age survivors of bacterial meningitis.* Acta Paediatrica, 2003. 92(2): p. 177-185.

89.   Grimwood, K., P. Anderson, V. Anderson, L. Tan, and T. Nolan, *Twelve year outcomes following bacterial meningitis: Further evidence for persisting effects.* Archives of Disease in Childhood, 2000. 83(2): p. 111-116.

Chapter 5

1.   Smith, A., *Breakfast cereal, caffeinated coffee, mood, and cognition.* Nutrition, 2000. 16(3): p. 228-229.

2.   Pollitt, E., S. Cueto, and E.R. Jacoby, *Fasting and cognition in well and undernourished schoolchildren: A review of three experimental studies.* American Journal of Clinical Nutrition, 1998. 67(4): p. 779s-784s.

3.   Simeon, D.T., and S.M. Grantham-McGregor, *Effects of missing breakfast on the cognitive functions of schoolchildren of differing nutritional status.* American Journal of Clinical Nutrition, 1989. 49(4): p. 646-653.

4.   Simeon, D.T., *School feeding in Jamaica: A review of its evaluation.* American Journal of Clinical Nutrition, 1998. 67(4): p. 790s-794s.

5.   Smith, A.P., *Stress, breakfast cereal consumption and cortisol.* Nutritional Neuroscience, 2002. 5(2): p. 141-144.

6.   Grantham-McGregor, S.M., S.M. Chang, and S.P. Walker, *Evaluation of school feeding programmes: Some Jamaican examples.* American Journal of Clinical Nutrition, 1998. 67(4): p. 785s-789s.

7.   Shariff, Z.M., J.T. Bond, and N.E. Johnson, *Nutrition and educational achievement of urban primary schoolchildren in Malaysia.* Asia Pacific Journal of Clinical Nutrition, 2000. 9(4): p. 264-273.

8.   Simeon, D., and S.M. Grantham-McGregor, *Nutritional deficiencies and children's behaviour and mental development.* Nutrition Research Reviews, 1990. 3: p. 1-24.

9.   Hutchinson, S.E., C.A. Powell, S.P. Walker, S.M. Chang, and S.M. Grantham-McGregor, *Nutrition, anaemia, geohelminth infection and school achievement in rural Jamaican primary schoolchildren.* European Journal of Clinical Nutrition, 1997. 51(11): p. 729-735.

10.   Partnership for Child Development, *An association between stunting and educational test scores in Vietnamese children.* 2000.

11.   Agarwal, K.N., D.K. Agarwal, and S.K. Upadhyay, *Impact of chronic undernutrition on higher mental functions in Indian boys aged 10-12 years.* Acta Paediatrica, 1995. 84(12): p. 1357-1361.

12.   Sigman, M., C. Neumann, A.A. Jansen, and N. Bwibo, *Cognitive abilities of Kenyan children in relation to nutrition, family characteristics, and education.* Child Development, 1989. 60(6): p. 1463-1474.

13.   Wachs, T.D., Z. Bishry, W. Moussa, F. Yunis, G. McCabe, G. Harrison, E. Sweifi, A. Kirksey, O. Galal, N. Jerome, F. Shaheen, *Nutritional intake and context as predictors of cognition and adaptive behaviour of Egyptian school-*

age children. International Journal of Behavioural Development, 1995. 18(3): p. 425-450.

14. McKay, H., L. Sinisterra, A. McKay, H. Gomez, and P. Lloreda, *Improving cognitive ability in chronically deprived children.* Science, 1978. 200(4339): p. 270-278.

15. Powell, C.A., S.P. Walker, S.M. Chang, and S.M. Grantham-McGregor, *Nutrition and education: A randomised trial of the effects of breakfast in rural primary schoolchildren.* American Journal of Clinical Nutrition, 1998. 68: p. 873-879.

16. Whaley, S.E., M. Sigman, C. Neumann, N. Bwibo, D. Guthrie, R.E. Weiss, S. Alber, and S.P. Murphy, *The impact of dietary intervention on the cognitive development of Kenyan schoolchildren.* Journal of Nutrition, 2003. 133(11): p. 3965S-3971S.

17. Grantham-McGregor, S.M., and C. Ani, *A review of studies on the effect of iron deficiency on cognitive development in children.* Journal of Nutrition, 2001. 131(2): p. 649S-666S.

18. Soemantri, A.G., E. Pollitt, and I. Kim, *Iron deficiency anaemia and educational achievement.* American Journal of Clinical Nutrition, 1985. 42(6): p. 1221-1228.

19. Seshadri, S., and T. Gopaldas, *Impact of iron supplementation on cognitive functions in preschool and school-aged children: The Indian experience.* American Journal of Clinical Nutrition, 1989. 50(3 Suppl): p. 675-684.

20. Pollitt, E., P. Hathirat, N.J. Kotchabhakdi, L. Missell, and A. Valyasevi, *Iron deficiency and educational achievement in Thailand.* American Journal of Clinical Nutrition, 1989. 50(3 Suppl): p. 687-696.

21. Azizi, F., A. Sarshar, M. Nafarabadi, A. Ghazi, M. Kimiagar, S. Noohi, N. Rahbar, A. Bahrami, and S. Kalantari, *Impairment of neuromotor and cognitive development in iodine deficient schoolchildren with normal physical growth.* Acta Endocrinologica, 1993. 129(6): p. 501-504.

22. Balogou, A.A.K., A. Doh, and K.E. Grunitzky, *Neurological disorders and endemic goitre: A comparative analysis of two districts of Togo.* Bulletin De La Societe De Pathologie Exotique, 2001. 94(5): p. 406-410.

23. Vermiglio, F., M. Sidoti, M.D. Finocchiaro, S. Battiato, V.P. Lopresti, S. Benvenga, and F. Trimarchi, *Defective neuromotor and cognitive ability in iodine deficient schoolchildren of an endemic goitre region in Sicily.* Journal of Clinical Endocrinology and Metabolism, 1990. 70(2): p. 379-384.

24. Huda, S.N., S.M. Grantham-McGregor, K.M. Rahman, and A. Tomkins, *Biochemical hypothyroidism secondary to iodine deficiency is associated with poor school achievement and cognition in Bangladeshi children.* Journal of Nutrition, 1999. 129(5): p. 980-987.

25. van den Briel, T., C.E. West, J. Hautvast, and E.A. Ategbo, *Mild iodine deficiency is associated with elevated hearing thresholds in children in Benin.* European Journal of Clinical Nutrition, 2001. 55(9): p. 763-768.

26. Huda, S.N., S.M. Grantham-McGregor, and A. Tomkins, *Cognitive and motor functions of iodine deficient but euthyroid children in Bangladesh do not benefit from iodised poppy seed oil (Lipiodol).* Journal of Nutrition, 2001. 131(1): p. 72-77.

27. van den Briel, T., C.E. West, N. Bleichrodt, F.J.R. van de Vijver, E.A. Ategbo, and J. Hautvast, *Improved iodine status is associated with improved mental performance of schoolchildren in Benin.* American Journal of Clinical Nutrition, 2000. 72(5): p. 1179-1185.

28.   Sandstead, H.H., J.G. Penland, N.W. Alcock, H. Hari, D. Xue, C. Chen, J.S. Li, F.
        Zhao, and J.J. Yang, *Effects of repletion with zinc and other micronutrients on
        neuropsychologic performance and growth of Chinese children.* American
        Journal of Clinical Nutrition, 1998. 68(2): p. 470S-475S.
29.   van Stuijvenberg, M.E., J.D. Kvalsvig, M. Faber, M. Kruger, D.G. Kenoyer, and
        A.J.S. Benade, *Effect of iron-, iodine-, and beta-carotene-fortified biscuits on
        the micronutrient status of primary schoolchildren: A randomised controlled
        trial.* American Journal of Clinical Nutrition, 1999. 69(3): p. 497-503.
30.   Vazir, S., B. Nagalla, V. Thangiah, V. Kamasamudram, and S. Bhattiprolu, *Effect
        of micronutrient supplement on health and nutritional status of
        schoolchildren: Mental function.* Nutrition, 2006. 22(1): p. S26-S32.
31.   Stephenson, L., *Impact of helminth infection on human nutrition.* 1987, London:
        Taylor and Francis.
32.   Mendez, M.A., and L.S. Adair, *Severity and timing of stunting in the first two
        years of life affect performance on cognitive tests in late childhood.* Journal of
        Nutrition, 1999. 129(8): p. 1555-1562.
33.   Watkins, W.E., and E. Pollitt, *Stupidity or worms: Do intestinal worms impair
        mental performance?* Psychological Bulletin, 1997. 121: p. 171-191.
34.   Jukes, M.C.H., C.A. Nokes, K.J. Alcock, J. Lambo, C. Kihamia, A. Mbise,
        L.W.E. Yona, L. Mwanri, A.M. Baddeley, A. Hall, and D.A.P. Bundy, *Heavy
        schistosomiasis associated with poor short-term memory and slower reaction
        times in Tanzanian schoolchildren.* Tropical Medicine and International
        Health, 2002. 7(2): p. 104-117.
35.   Nokes, C., S.T. McGarvey, L. Shiue, G. Wu, H. Wu, D.A.P. Bundy, and G.R.
        Olds, *Evidence for an improvement in cognitive function following treatment
        of Schistosoma japonicum infection in Chinese primary schoolchildren.*
        American Journal of Tropical Medicine and Hygiene, 1999. 60(4): p. 556-
        565.
36.   Simeon, D.T., S.M. Grantham-McGregor, and M.S. Wong, *Trichuris trichiura
        infection and cognition in children: Results of a randomised clinical trial.*
        Parasitology, 1995. 110(Pt 4): p. 457-464.
37.   Simeon, D.T., S.M. Grantham-McGregor, J.E. Callender, and M.S. Wong,
        *Treatment of Trichuris trichiura infections improves growth, spelling scores
        and school attendance in some children.* Journal of Nutrition, 1995. 125(7): p.
        1875-1883.
38.   Sternberg, R.J., C. Powell, P. McGrane, and S.M. Grantham-McGregor, *Effects of
        a parasitic infection on cognitive functioning.* Journal of Experimental
        Psychology-Applied, 1997. 3(1): p. 67-76.
39.   Grigorenko, E., R. Sternberg, D. Ngorosho, C. Nokes, M.C.H. Jukes, K.J. Alcock,
        J. Lambo, and D.A.P. Bundy, *Effects of antiparasitic treatment on
        dynamically and statically tested cognitive skills over time.* Journal of Applied
        Developmental Psychology, 2006. 27: p. 499-526.
40.   Fernando, D., D. De Silva, R. Carter, K.N. Mendis, and R. Wickremasinghe, *A
        randomised, double-blind, placebo-controlled, clinical trial of the impact of
        malaria prevention on the educational attainment of schoolchildren.*
        American Journal of Tropical Medicine and Hygiene, 2006. 74(3): p. 386-
        393.
41.   Clarke, S.E., J.K. Njagi, M.C.H. Jukes, B.B.A. Estambale, L. Khasakhala, A.
        Ajanga, J. Otido, S. Ochola, S. Brooker, and P. Magnussen, *Intermittent*

preventive treatment in schools: Effects on malaria parasitaemia, anaemia and school performance, in prep.

42. Cohen, S., and A. Smith, *Psychology of common colds and other infections,* in *Viral and other infections of the human respiratory tract,* S. Myint and D. Taylor-Robinson, Editors. 1996, Chapman and Hall.

43. Wolters, P.L., P. Brouwers, H.A. Moss, and P.A. Pizzo, *Differential receptive and expressive language functioning of children with symptomatic HIV disease and relation to CT scan brain abnormalities.* Pediatrics, 1995. 95(1): p. 112-119.

44. Frank, E.G., G.M. Foley, and A. Kuchuk, *Cognitive functioning in school-age children with human immunodeficiency virus.* Perceptual and Motor Skills, 1997. 85(1): p. 267-272.

45. Pizzo, P.A., J. Eddy, J. Falloon, F.M. Balis, R.F. Murphy, H. Moss, P. Wolters, P. Brouwers, P. Jarosinski, M. Rubin, S. Broder, R. Yarchoan, A. Brunetti, M. Maha, S. Nusinofflehrman, and D.G. Poplack, *Effect of continuous intravenous-infusion of Zidovudine (Azt) in children with symptomatic HIV infection.* New England Journal of Medicine, 1988. 319(14): p. 889-896.

46. Wolters, P.L., P. Brouwers, H.A. Moss, and P.A. Pizzo, *Adaptive-behaviour of children with symptomatic HIV infection before and after Zidovudine therapy.* Journal of Pediatric Psychology, 1994. 19(1): p. 47-61.

47. Stolar, A., and F. Fernandez, *Psychiatric perspective of paediatric human immunodeficiency virus infection.* Southern Medical Journal, 1997. 90(10): p. 1007-1016.

48. Brady, M.T., N. McGrath, P. Brouwers, R. Gelber, M.G. Fowler, R. Yogev, N. Hutton, Y.J. Bryson, C.D. Mitchell, S. Fikrig, *et al., Randomised study of the tolerance and efficacy of high- versus low-dose Zidovudine in human immunodeficiency virus-infected children with mild to moderate symptoms (AIDS clinical trials group 128).* Journal of Infectious Diseases, 1996. 173(5): p. 1097-1106.

49. Brivio, L., R. Tornaghi, L. Musetti, P. Marchisio, and N. Principi, *Improvement of auditory brain-stem responses after treatment with Zidovudine in a child with AIDS.* Pediatric Neurology, 1991. 7(1): p. 53-55.

50. Brouwers, P., C. Decarli, G. Tudorwilliams, L. Civitello, H. Moss, and P.A. Pizzo, *Interrelations among patterns of change in neurocognitive, CT brain imaging and CD4 measures associated with antiretroviral therapy in children with symptomatic HIV infection.* Advances in Neuroimmunology, 1994. 4(3): p. 223-231.

51. Moss, H.A., P. Brouwers, P.L. Wolters, L. Wiener, S. Hersh, and P.A. Pizzo, *The development of a Q-Sort behavioural rating procedure for paediatric HIV patients.* Journal of Pediatric Psychology, 1994. 19(1): p. 27-46.

52. Makame, V., C. Ani, and S.M. Grantham-McGregor, *Psychological well-being of orphans in Dar Es Salaam, Tanzania.* Acta Paediatrica, 2002. 91(4): p. 459-465.

53. Nyamukapa, C.A., S. Gregson, B. Lopman, S. Saito, H.J. Watts, R. Monasch, and M.C.H. Jukes, *HIV-associated orphanhood and children's psychosocial disorders: Theoretical framework tested with data from Zimbabwe,* in press. American Journal of Public Health.

54. Bhargava, A., *AIDS epidemic and the psychological well-being and school participation of Ethiopian orphans.* Psychology, Health and Medicine, 2005. 10(3): p. 263-275.

55.   Nokes, C., S.M. Grantham-McGregor, A.W. Sawyer, E.S. Cooper, B.A. Robinson, and D.A.P. Bundy, *Moderate to heavy infections of Trichuris trichiura affect cognitive function in Jamaican schoolchildren.* Parasitology, 1992. 104(Pt 3): p. 539-547.

Chapter 6

1.   Guyatt, H., *The cost of delivering and sustaining a control programme for schistosomiasis and soil-transmitted helminthiasis.* Acta Tropica, 2003. 86(2-3): p. 267-274.
2.   Del Rosso, J.M., *School feeding programmes: Improving effectiveness and increasing benefit to education.* 1999, Partnership for Child Development: London.
3.   Partnership for Child Development, *The cost of large-scale school health programmes which deliver anthelminthics to children in Ghana and Tanzania.* Acta Tropica, 1999. 73: p. 183-204.
4.   Bobadilla, J.L., P. Cowley, P. Musgrove, and H. Saxenian., *The essential package of services in developing countries,* in *Population Health and Nutrition Background Paper Series.* 1994, The World Bank: Washington DC.
5.   Murray, C., and A. Lopez, eds. *The global burden of disease: Global burden of disease and injury series. Volume I.* 1996, Harvard University Press: Boston: Harvard School of Public Health.
6.   Psacharopoulos, G., and M. Woodhall, *Education for development: An analysis of investment choices.* 1985, New York: Oxford University Press.
7.   Strauss, J., and D. Thomas, *Human resources: Empirical modelling of household and family decisions.,* in *Handbook of Development Economics,* J. Behrman and T.N. Srinivasan, Editors. 1995, Elsevier: Amsterdam.
8.   Jamison, D., and Lawrence J. Lau, *Farmer education and farm efficiency.* 1982, The World Bank: Baltimore.
9.   Card, D., *Estimating the return to schooling: Progress on some persistent econometric problems.* Econometrica, 2001. 69(5): p. 1127-1160.
10.   Miguel, E., and M. Kremer, *Worms: Identifying impacts on education and health in the presence of treatment externalities.* Econometrica, 2004. 72(1): p. 159-217.
11.   Zax, J.S., and D.I. Rees, *IQ, academic performance, environment, and earnings.* Review of Economics and Statistics, 2002. 84(4): p. 600-616.
12.   Hanushek, E.A., and L. Wosman, *The role of education quality for economic growth,* in *Policy Research Working Paper.* 2007, The World Bank: Washington, DC. p. 94.
13.   Simeon, D.T., and S.M. Grantham-McGregor, *Effects of missing breakfast on the cognitive functions of schoolchildren of differing nutritional status.* American Journal of Clinical Nutrition, 1989. 49(4): p. 646-653.
14.   Soemantri, A.G., E. Pollitt, and I. Kim, *Iron deficiency anaemia and educational achievement.* American Journal of Clinical Nutrition, 1985. 42(6): p. 1221-1228.
15.   Nokes, C., S.M. Grantham-McGregor, A.W. Sawyer, E.S. Cooper, B.A. Robinson, and D.A.P. Bundy, *Moderate to heavy infections of Trichuris trichiura affect cognitive function in Jamaican schoolchildren.* Parasitology, 1992. 104(Pt 3): p. 539-547.

16.   Grigorenko, E., R.J. Sternberg, D. Ngorosho, C. Nokes, M.C.H. Jukes, K.J. Alcock, J. Lambo, and D.A.P. Bundy, *Effects of antiparasitic treatment on dynamically and statically tested cognitive skills over time.* Journal of Applied Developmental Psychology, 2006. 27: p. 499-526.

17.   Liddell, C., and G. Rae, *Predicting early grade retention: A longitudinal investigation of primary school progress in a sample of rural South African children.* British Journal of Educational Psychology, 2001. 71: p. 413-428.

18.   Jukes, M.C.H., C.A. Nokes, K.J. Alcock, J. Lambo, C. Kihamia, A. Mbise, L.W.E. Yona, L. Mwanri, A.M. Baddeley, A. Hall, and D.A.P. Bundy, *Heavy schistosomiasis associated with poor short-term memory and slower reaction times in Tanzanian schoolchildren.* Tropical Medicine and International Health, 2002. 7(2): p. 104-117.

19.   Moll, P.G., *Primary schooling, cognitive skills and wages in South Africa.* Economica, 1998. 65(258): p. 263-284.

20.   Jukes, M.C.H., M. Pinder, E.L. Grigorenko, H.B. Smith, G. Walraven, E.M. Bariau, R.J. Sternberg, L.J. Drake, P. Milligan, Y.B. Cheung, B.M. Greenwood, D.A.P. Bundy*, Long-term impact of malaria chemoprophylaxis on cognitive abilities and educational attainment: Follow-up of a controlled trial.* PLoS Clinical Trials, 2006. 1(4): p. e19.

21.   UNESCO, *EFA Global Monitoring Report 2003/4: Gender and Education for All. The leap to equality.* 2003, UNESCO: Paris.

22.   American Psychiatric Association, *Diagnostic and statistical manual of mental disorders (4th ed.).* 1994, Washington, DC.

23.   Pritchett, L., and D. Filmer, *What education production functions really show: A positive theory of education expenditures.* Economics of Education Review, 1999. 18(2): p. 223-239.

24.   Kremer, M., *Randomised evaluations of educational programmes in developing countries: Some lessons.* American Economic Review, 2003. 93(2): p. 102-106.

25.   Lockheed, M.E., and A.M. Verspoor, *Improving primary education in developing countries.* 1991, Oxford: Oxford University Press for The World Bank.

26.   Morley, S., and D. Coady, *From social assistance to social development: Targeting educational subsidies in developing countries.* 2003, Washington, DC: Centre for Global Development/International Food Policy Research Institute.

Chapter 7

1.   Karoly, L.A., P. Greenwood, W.S.S. Everinghma, J. Hoube, R. Kilburn, M.P. Rydell, C.M. Sanders, and J. Chiesa, *Investing in our children: What we know and what we don't know about the costs and benefits of early childhood interventions.* 1998, Santa Monica, CA: RAND. 159.

2.   WHO. *Integrated Management of Childhood Illness.* 2006, Available from: http://www.who.int/child-adolescent-health/publications/pubIMCI.htm.

3.   De Silva, N., S. Brooker, P. Hotez, A. Montresor, D. Engels, and L. Savioli, *Soil-transmitted helminth infections: Updating the global picture.* Trends in Parasitology, forthcoming, 2003.

4.   Filmer, D., and L. Pritchett, *The effect of household wealth on educational attainment: Evidence from 35 countries.* Population and Development Review, 1999. 25(1).
5.   World Bank, The FRESH framework: A toolkit for task managers. Human development network. 2000, The World Bank: Washington DC.
6.   Warren, K.S., D.A.P. Bundy, R.M. Anderson, A.R. Davis, D.A. Henderson, D.T. Jamison and others. *Helminth infection* in *Disease control priorities in developing countries,* ed. D.T. Jamison, W.H. Mosley, A.R. Measham and J.L. Bobadilla. 1993, Oxford University Press: New York.
7.   UNESCO, *The Dakar Framework for Action: Education for All – Meeting our collective commitments.* 2000, UNESCO: World Education Forum, Dakar.

Index